Scoliosis does not Hurt

A Healthcare Journey

June Parker

Copyright © 2022 June Parker
http://www.scoliosisdoesnothurt.com/

All rights reserved.
In accordance with the U.S. Copyright Act of 1976, the scanning, uploading, and electronic sharing of any part of this book without the permission of the publisher/author constitute unlawful piracy and theft of the author's intellectual property.

If you would like to use material from the book (except for review purposes), prior written permission must be obtained by contacting the author at june.sdnh@gmail.com. Thank you for your support of author's rights.

Cover picture courtesy of Shutterstock

ISBN: 9798409941871

Table of Contents

ONE: Discovery 1

TWO: Scoliosis Does Not Hurt 9

THREE: The Beginning 17

FOUR: Dr. Wong 23

FIVE: The Paper Tickers 31

SIX: Is Anybody Listening 41

SEVEN: Where's Morgan 47

EIGHT: Strawberry, Blueberry and Green Apple 57

NINE: The Shopping Cart 65

TEN: Third Times a Charm 73

ELEVEN: My Turn 83

TWELVE: Only Three Rides 89

THIRTEEN: Are We Missing Something? 97

FOURTEEN: Dealing with the Wait 101

FIFTEEN: Spinal Fusion 105

SIXTEEN: Pain Girl 115

SEVENTEEN: Dad's Fed Up 123

EIGHTEEN: Drama Queen 133

NINETEEN: The Ambulance is on its Way 139

TWENTY: Spine Surgery Number Four 147

*This book is dedicated to Morgan,
may your strength carry you through the next chapters of
your life.*

Veni vidi vici

ONE

DISCOVERY

The end of grade five was upon us and we had such an incredible summer planned. We revelled in the fact that private school seemed to be exactly what Morgan needed to succeed.

After school had ended in the summer of 2006, we headed to Victoria, British Columbia. Arguably, Victoria is one of the most beautiful cities in Canada. We were from land locked Alberta and were so excited to be near the Pacific Ocean. Of course, we took this opportunity to avail ourselves of the Whale Watching Tours.

We sped away towards an area where whales are known to frequent and sure enough, we saw whales. I wouldn't say up close and personal, as laws that govern these tour boats ensured that we were not too close. On the way back to land the tour guide screamed "Minke.... minke...these are my favourite types of whales." We had never heard of the minke whale, but the tour guide did tell us that they were one of the smallest known whales. He continued to explain that they migrated to the coast of British Columbia in the spring and returned south to warmer waters in the fall. To be honest, I think he was just trying to get the crowd excited about these small whales as we were not able to get a good view of the larger whales, which was the point of the tour.

The next day, we rented a car and headed north on Vancouver Island where we knew we had to take in the West Coast Trail. There definitely was a lot of history along this trail and there were gentle reminders of the first settlers who had explored and used this trail as a part of their everyday lives. Parks Canada indicates that the trail is 75 km or 46.5 miles long while many hikers feel that it is quite a bit longer. We had no intention of walking the whole trail, we definitely were not a family of hikers, but we did want to walk on it, explore it and to view and listen to the ocean while we were there.

The beauty is beyond breathtaking and just listening to the ocean as it slapped against the huge rocks was such an amazing experience. Morgan was very excited with how huge the trees and the size of the leaves were. We did not have trees like this in Southern Alberta, this truly was a wonderful experience. We were having such a great time; we brought a picnic lunch and thoroughly enjoyed the whole adventure.

Morgan, however, was starting to complain that she couldn't walk too far. We were aware of the fact that Morgan had difficulty walking far. She was eleven years old, and we knew that for whatever reason, none medically, we were assured of that, she couldn't walk far and we knew that whatever we did we would only be able to go a limited distance.

I knew that we had done everything humanly possible to get to the bottom of why Morgan could only walk so far, but healthcare professionals kept reassuring us that nothing was wrong. I didn't want to ruin our beautiful vacation on Vancouver Island by focusing on a negative issue. Morgan enjoyed the trail and loved everything about being on the west coast of Canada.

The next day, before heading back to Calgary, we visited the parliament buildings in Victoria. These majestic buildings were built in the late 1800's and the architectural beauty was indescribable. In this area there were flags and monuments of each province, so we took pictures of each other near the respective province that we were born in. Morgan stood proudly by the Ontario flag and monument, Scott by the Saskatchewan flag and monument and I stood by the distinctive Quebec flag and monument.

The following weekend we were back in Alberta where we have lived since shortly after Morgan's birth. We were boating and fishing on McGregor Lake. McGregor Lake was originally a man-made reservoir serving the agricultural communities in the area.

McGregor Lake is in Vulcan County, between the small communities of Vulcan and Lomond.

It was a beautiful day and Scott was captaining the boat with Morgan on a tube. She was screaming with excitement. She was having so much fun and didn't want Scott to stop.

She screamed "Faster Daddy faster!" at each turn. Scott was whipping the tube pretty good, but the look on Morgan's face was something I will never forget. She was a very excited little girl enjoying the water with her Mom and Dad and all those pesky problems that nagged Morgan were now behind us, it was as if she didn't have a care in the world.

Morgan was suddenly thrown off the tube and was in the middle of the lake. She did have her life vest on so there was no concern of her drowning, but she shouted out that her leg hurt from the fall. The hazard of tubing is what I thought as I massaged her leg.

A few days later, Morgan mentioned that her upper back hurt. We were now living in Springbank Hill, a community in the southwest part of Calgary, and I was working from home with a successful mortgage broker. Morgan had googled information online and told me that she thought that she had scoliosis.

I was super busy that day and had difficulty holding back my laughter. What an imagination my daughter had. I couldn't believe that she would think that she had scoliosis, how ridiculous. I told her to take a couple of over-the-counter pain medicine and that the pain would subside.

The following week, we were off to visit my brother and his family in Newmarket, Ontario. We had so much planned for the short visit. On the plane ride, Morgan again mentioned that her upper back hurt. It was late July by this time, and I was growing concerned that her back pain had persisted for over a month. I made a mental note to contact her pediatrician, Dr. Wong, when we got back.

It was great visiting with my brother and his family, they made us feel welcomed. I so appreciated Morgan having an opportunity to get to know my side of the family.

We did travel back to Quebec most summers to visit with my family there, but now we were visiting my brother and his family in Newmarket. Our plans to visit Canada's Wonderland were squashed as Morgan said that she could not do that much walking because of the pain in her back.

I encouraged my brother to go ahead with his family, Morgan and I sat the trip out. Without a doubt, my concern about this back pain grew. What kid would travel halfway across the country and not want to go to Canada's Wonderland?

We no sooner arrived at home in Calgary when Morgan got a call from her good friend Miranda asking her to go with her to her family's cabin in Northern Alberta. I overheard the conversation and when Morgan replied that she would go, I was relieved as it made me feel as if her back pain wasn't that bad.

However, on her way out the door she yelled "Mom, don't forget to call Dr. Wong, I want an appointment the day I get back as this back pain is horrible." So much for her having forgotten about the back pain.

I called Dr. Wong's office and his receptionist, that I now knew quite well, surprised me by saying that he was out of the office for an undetermined amount of time as he had cancer. "Cancer" I repeated to his receptionist, and she replied yes, he had a growth on his spine. I would be lying if I said that my mind did not go there with Morgan's back issue.

I never thought of something like that. Was it a possibility? Could she have a tumour on her spine like Dr. Wong did?

I knew that I was getting ahead of myself, but Morgan was able to handle pain very well. But this back pain was different. I watched as she somehow managed to cut the circumference of her leg in the hot tub but didn't want to stop to have me take a look at it.

I watched as she went down a hill on her bicycle and flipped, leaving the imprint of the handlebars on her stomach and she walked it off. I watched as she tripped over a tree root that was sticking out of the ground and did a faceplant and wanted to go on. She was never one to complain about her injuries.

She had since age five complained of hip pain and complained that she couldn't walk too far, but she was able to endure pain and had no time for self pity. This certainly was not Morgan. She was not a complainer, and she could handle pain, so of course my thoughts did go there.

The receptionist then told me that there was one paediatrician that worked part time to replace Dr. Wong and she was only able to book me an appointment in late August.

That was a full three weeks away. I was always able to get in to see Dr. Wong the same week at the very latest. This was due to the fact that Dr. Wong was familiar with Morgan's many health issues and always tried to accommodate us. I wasn't used to waiting three weeks to see Morgan's doctor.

Hearing the news about Dr. Wong was heartbreaking. Our whole family recognized him as an integral part of Morgan's well being. We valued and respected him not only as Morgan's doctor, but he was forever intertwined with our family. His words and the fact that he genuinely cared made such a difference for us.

We met with Dr. Wong's replacement, and she seemed to be so patient and understanding. We told her about what had transpired over the summer, our trip to Victoria, the boating at McGregor Lake and our time in Newmarket.

The Paediatrician asked Morgan where her pain was and Morgan demonstrated that the pain was in the upper left quadrant of her back. She asked Morgan to bend over and to lift her t-shirt up in the back. Morgan bent over and I was overcome with shock.

I could not believe my eyes. She had a huge hump on her upper left side, and it was so visible when the doctor had Morgan bend over so that she could take a look at it. She told us immediately that Morgan had scoliosis and that she thought it was severe based on the deformity that had already set in.

Morgan, still relatively young at 11, could only think to say "See I told you Mom that I had scoliosis!" I was still in a state of shock and could see by the look on the doctor's face that this was serious.

The doctor instructed us to get an x-ray immediately and that she was going to be contacting the orthopedic unit to let them know about Morgan. She felt confident that with the results of the x-ray that Morgan would be seen quickly.

Morgan and I got into the car, and I called Scott to let him know that we were going for a rush x-ray because Morgan had scoliosis.

I have no idea what Scott's response was as I couldn't process the whole scene. I couldn't wrap my head around the fact that less than an hour ago a doctor showed me that my daughter had severe scoliosis and we were now headed to get a rush x-ray. I have no idea which roads we took or how long it took us to get there. I was just driving with a single purpose, to get the x-ray.

The beauty with the innocence of a child, here I was trying to appear calm so as to not upset Morgan, and she seemed calm and kept repeating "I told you I had scoliosis." Believe me, I was far from calm.

I'm not sure that everything had sunk in yet for her. I'm not sure she realized that Dr. Wong's replacement had sent us to get a rush x-ray and that she was being immediately referred to the orthopaedic unit. I'm not sure what she understood at this point, I wasn't really sure what I did either.

The next day the phone rang. I looked and noticed that it was Dr. Wong's office, obviously not Dr. Wong himself, as he wasn't in the office, but his replacement. I was on the main level of our house in Springbank Hill and Morgan was in the basement. I did not want her to hear what was being said, so I rushed up the stairs into the master bedroom and closed the door behind me.

The doctor told me that Morgan had serious scoliosis that required that she be seen by an orthopaedic surgeon immediately. She continued to say that Morgan had a left side curve that measured 52 degrees.

Of course, all of this was foreign to me. I detected a sense of urgency from this doctor. She did tell me that left side curves are not common and that at the level of curvature there is concern for her heart.

She said that most orthopaedic surgeons consider surgery at the 40 – 45-degree mark. I am sure that she told me more than this, but this is all I was able to grasp and able to retain.

I've often heard of the expression 'paralyzed in fear' and thought that it was such an odd saying. I mean normally with fear you want to run, not stay in the same place. I truly understood the meaning of 'paralyzed in fear' because I certainly was.

I hung up from speaking with the doctor and I literally could not move. I wanted to scream. I wanted the whole world to know how unfair this was. I could not. I was paralyzed in fear.

Once the initial shock wore off, I jumped under the covers and cried. I couldn't believe it.

I wanted to call Scott and let him know what the doctor had told me, but I couldn't. I could not come to terms with things. I did not want to call Scott at work and have everyone hear his wife being hysterical. I knew that I needed to calm down before calling him.

I'm not sure how long I stayed under the covers. It was longer than 10 minutes, it could even have been half an hour. In my despair, I was losing the concept of time.

I knew that I wanted to call Scott before I spoke with Morgan. I knew that I had to let him know as soon as possible, as he was as anxious as I was about the results of Morgan's x-ray.

Scott could tell that I had been crying and he did his best to comfort me considering that we were speaking with each other via cell phone. I knew Scott was in shock. I knew that it was difficult for him. Now, I had to go tell Morgan.

She was only eleven years old, by now, she knew more about scoliosis than I did. She knew she had scoliosis when I doubted her.

I doubted her because there is no scoliosis in either Scott's family or mine, it's that simple. I never knew anyone that had had scoliosis and had limited understanding of it.

I decided that I would tell her that indeed she did have scoliosis. Although the doctor had confirmed this the previous day. I would not share with her the degree of the curve, as I could pretend that I didn't know. Nor would I tell her that it was a left side curve, even though her pain was on her left side, and she probably could figure this out. I didn't want to give her more information than I had to as I knew that she would be researching everything.

I was just going to tell her that she had scoliosis and that we would soon be meeting with an orthopaedic specialist. I did not want to use the word surgeon, not sure if this was for her benefit or mine.

The appointment with the orthopaedic surgeon was scheduled for the following week. Scott and I knew that the situation had to be serious for Morgan to be seen so quickly. In the meantime, I wanted to learn as much as I could about scoliosis.

I was feeling horrible because I was angry that Dr. Wong wasn't there to help me understand what Morgan was going through. Dr. Wong was there every step of the way, he had been there through all 10 ear surgeries, he had been my rock. I counted on Dr. Wong; he was always there. I needed him to be there, but he was fighting cancer, how horribly selfish of me. I felt so ashamed.

I needed to forget about Dr. Wong. He would have been there if he could. I had to focus on Morgan, and I had to try to understand as much as I could before the appointment.

I wasn't sure what I would be told. I knew it wouldn't be good and I knew it would be scary. It was far worse than I ever imagined.

TWO

SCOLIOSIS DOES NOT HURT

One of the first things I discovered while doing research is that the word scoliosis was derived from the Greek word skoliosis which literally means "crookedness".

Of course, discovering that scoliosis was derived from a Greek word brought me back to an incredibly funny quote from the movie My Big Fat Greek Wedding. One of my favourite Gus Portokalos quotes: "Give me a word, any word, and I will show you how the root of that word is Greek!"

Movie quotes aside, the Mayo Clinic's website states that:

"Scoliosis is a sideways curvature of the spine that occurs most often during the growth spurt just before puberty. While scoliosis can be caused by conditions such as cerebral palsy and muscular dystrophy, the cause of most scoliosis is unknown. About 3% of adolescents have scoliosis.

Most cases of scoliosis are mild, but some spine deformities continue to get more severe as children grow. Severe scoliosis can be disabling. An especially severe spinal curve can reduce the amount of space within the chest, making it difficult for the lungs to function properly.

Children who have mild scoliosis are monitored closely, usually with X-rays, to see if the curve is getting worse. In many cases, no treatment is necessary. Some children will need to wear a brace to stop the curve from worsening. Others may need surgery to keep the scoliosis from worsening and to straighten severe cases of scoliosis."[1]

I read over the paragraph that states "Most cases of scoliosis are mild, but some spine deformities continue to get more severe as children grow. Severe scoliosis can be disabling."

I didn't want to let that sink in. I didn't want to admit that although we hadn't met with the orthopaedic surgeon yet, Dr. Wong's replacement had already told me several times that Morgan had severe scoliosis.

Of course, I couldn't stop there. I had to find out more about a left side curve, as the doctor seemed quite concerned about this. I referred to many articles and websites, but this article on the website of Medical News Today really put a fear into what a left side curve meant.

"Levoscoliosis, which involves a left spinal curve, is less common than scoliosis that involves a right spinal curve. In fact, a 2014 review estimated that 85 – 90 % of adolescents with scoliosis had right curves.

Health professionals consider levoscoliosis to be a particularly dangerous form of scoliosis because the heart is located in the left side of the body. Also, levoscoliosis is more likely to be linked to other conditions — including spinal tumors, growths, and neuromuscular disorders — than scoliosis with a right curvature."[2]

At this point, I was ready to throw up. I was overwhelmed. I was frightened and very angry that we didn't discover this sooner. There were signs, yet they were ignored. Not by me, but by professionals. I feel incredibly guilty, could I have done more? Why didn't I notice that she had scoliosis?

---

[1] *https://www.mayoclinic.org/diseases-conditions/scoliosis/symptoms-causes/syc-20350716*

[2] *https://www.medicalnewstoday.com/articles/320207*

Of course, I googled symptoms. I googled everything about scoliosis, and I researched many websites, read many books and I still felt as if I did not know enough about it. However according to the website Treating Scoliosis," catching scoliosis early is critical because once a curve measures 25 degrees or more, there is a 68 percent chance scoliosis may get worse. You may detect signs of mild idiopathic scoliosis in its early stages by observing five different points on your child's body.

Eye line Are your child's eyes level or is the eye line tilted?

Shoulder level Do your child's shoulders hang evenly or is one higher than the other?

Hips Are your child's hips even or is one hip higher or more pronounced?

Forward head posture When you look from the side, does your child's mid-ear line up with the tip of the shoulder?

Head to hip line Would a line from the center of your child's eyes line up horizontally to the center of the hips."[3]

As I reviewed these points listed on the Treating Scoliosis website, I knew that Morgan was already well beyond the 25-degree curve, her curve was more than double that. I believed that I was ready for the appointment with the orthopedic surgeon. But in my heart, I knew that I was no way ready. When you put emotion into a health condition, there is no way that you could ever be prepared for such an appointment.

We met the orthopaedic surgeon. At this point, Morgan was still on a high because, as she put it "I knew that I had Scoliosis!" I, however, am terrified, plain and simple.

The surgeon seemed so understanding and he was so calm and reassuring. I felt better listening to him, he had a Dr. Wong type of personality and I appreciated him for that. His nurse

---

[3] https://www.treatingscoliosis.com/what-is-scoliosis/

seemed efficient, but without a doubt, she did not have the personality that the surgeon did.

Morgan, having done significantly more research about scoliosis, bounced in place while announcing to the surgeon "I need surgery... right?" The surgeon was impressed with her vibrant personality and said that he felt certain that she needed surgery, but that he wanted to check out a few things first. He told Morgan that once she had surgery that it would be as if she never had scoliosis at all.

He continued to go on to explain to us that he felt that Morgan had idiopathic scoliosis. Idiopathic simply refers to the fact that the medical community had no real understanding of why an individual has scoliosis. I questioned this. I was not holding anything back. I did not think that Morgan had idiopathic scoliosis. I believed that everything that Morgan had gone through up to this discovery pointed to her having scoliosis.

I told the surgeon of Morgan's past medical issues and concerns. I wasn't comfortable with just labeling Morgan's scoliosis as idiopathic in nature. I wanted to get to the root of everything. I needed an answer. I needed him to understand what Morgan had been through.

I was so used to being ignored by health care professionals. I wasn't going to take it anymore.

The surgeon seemed to dismiss what I was saying. However, he ordered a brain MRI due to the fact that it was a left side curve. Sometimes when there is a tumour on the brain it can cause left side scoliosis.

Perfect, just perfect, a brain MRI, there could be a tumour on her brain! I had to be stoic. I did not want Morgan to see concern on my face or hear it in my voice.

She was just 11 years old; how could she understand any of this? I was having difficulty processing it myself.

The nurse asked if she could take a photo of Morgan and me together so that should we call, she would remember who we were. I had never heard of this before. Was this good? Was this bad? I had no idea. I had too much to deal with to protest, so she took the photo, and we left.

On the car ride home, I was holding back my tears. I couldn't allow Morgan to see how upset or concerned I was.

Morgan could feel my stress and said "Mom, don't worry, the surgeon promised that after surgery it will be as if I never had scoliosis at all." I desperately wanted to believe these words.

As I discussed the potential tumour on the brain scenario with Scott, I couldn't hold back my tears. As always, Scott was strong, and he was reassuring and way more logical than I could be. He said that we shouldn't be upset yet. We had no idea if she had a tumour or not. I was making myself sick with worry.

The day after our appointment was the start of grade six. I was happy that Morgan had something other than scoliosis to focus on. She had a new teacher who seemed nice and understanding. I explained about Morgan's scoliosis and that she would be needing surgery. I wanted to be sure that the teacher understood Morgan's emotional state. A few weeks later, we were sitting in the waiting area of the imaging department for the brain MRI. I felt that Morgan wasn't concerned about it or the reasoning behind it. I'm not sure that she heard or understood what the surgeon had said.

Perhaps it just made me feel better that I believed that she didn't understand. I used this time to make light of the situation. I jokingly said to her that the surgeon was checking to see if she had any brains. We both laughed and at that moment, laughter was what we needed.

Morgan, unlike me, was unphased by the brain MRI. I knew waiting for results would be difficult. I told myself that worrying wouldn't change anything. Yet, I was her mom, and I couldn't help but worry.

At our second appointment with the orthopaedic surgeon, we were told that the MRI scan was fine, whatever fine really meant. I had to stop and acknowledge to myself that this was a victory, no tumour of any kind. At this point, I had become jaded by the entire health care journey I had been on with my daughter.

I asked the orthopaedic surgeon when the surgery would be scheduled. He went on to say that there were many children that required this surgery, and that Morgan would be put on the list. He added that Morgan would be evaluated on a monthly basis and after each appointment, a decision would be made as to where she would land on the waiting list.

I was appalled. I couldn't believe that in Canada children would be treated this way. We tell them that they require a major invasive surgery, but we have no clue when that surgery will be.

That we leave families hanging with this information and not having a date for surgery was inconceivable to me. We needed to know, to get prepared. If that were even possible.

How did they expect families to deal with the anxiety and frustration of not having a date for surgery? This seemed to make matters even worse.

We were conditioned to wait for health care services, like all Canadians, but this went above and beyond.

Overwhelmed, disappointed, frustrated, stressed don't even begin to describe how I was feeling. I needed to speak with Dr. Wong about the situation, I needed his input. I needed his guidance, but he was in a fight of his own.

How could I be so selfish? Dr. Wong is an incredible paediatrician, a wonderful human being and I was worried about me and my daughter. I told myself to get over it. I knew that any doctor that Dr. Wong chose to replace him would be a good doctor. I had confidence in that.

When I called to see if I could meet with one of Dr. Wong's replacements, I was told that the earliest appointment would be in two months. Yes, two months. I was used to seeing Dr. Wong the same week. I would have to wait two months to see a replacement paediatrician.

Morgan came to me a few weeks later and started talking about the pain she was feeling and the anxiety of not knowing when the surgery would be. I wanted to hug her and take away all the pain. I wanted to tell her it would all be over soon but how could I lie to my daughter?

Scoliosis Does Not Hurt

I contacted the orthopaedic surgeon's office and spoke with the efficient nurse that took our photo. I mentioned to her that Morgan was having difficulty in gym class because she felt more pain in her upper back with the exercises and/or sport activities.

To my complete and utter surprise, she screamed into the phone "SCOLIOSIS DOES NOT HURT!" I could not believe what I was hearing. This nurse was an older woman with years of experience in the orthopaedic unit, how could she say that scoliosis did not hurt?

I tried to interject and let her know that the only way that we had discovered that Morgan had scoliosis was due to the pain. I did go on a tangent about everything that we had been through to finally get the diagnosis of scoliosis. Now, we needed some help, some guidance and Morgan's paediatrician was unavailable because he was fighting cancer.

She did not like a parent challenging her and her voice went up an octave or two and screamed "DO I HAVE TO REPEAT MYSELF; SCOLIOSIS DOES NOT HURT!"

I was so upset by her comment and so emotionally invested in my daughter's health care that I could feel my voice trembling. I did not want it to tremble. I knew that I had to be strong, perhaps even forceful, but emotions got the best of me. I knew that there was nothing that I could have said that would have changed this woman's mind, even though the only way that we discovered Morgan's scoliosis was due to the pain.

With my voice still trembling, I asked if she or the surgeon could refer Morgan to a paediatrician as Dr. Wong was away indefinitely fighting cancer and two months seemed too long to wait.

She lost it, totally lost it she was so upset with me and yelled "YOU OBVIOUSLY DON'T UNDERSTAND THE HEALTH CARE SYSTEM, PAEDIATRICIANS REFER PATIENTS TO US, WE DO NOT REFER PATIENTS TO PAEDIATRICIANS."

I had enough of listening to this rude and insensitive nurse. It was obvious that I would have to keep fighting. I wondered when did the fighting stop? When was enough enough? Why did I have to continuously fight?

The words of the MLA that I had spoken with years earlier were coming back to me "Health care first and foremost is for the most vulnerable in our society." Bullshit! I thought long and hard and wondered what I should do. I couldn't give up, Morgan still needed me to fight for her. There was no way around that nurse in the orthopaedic unit, she was the gatekeeper.

In order to understand our journey in the healthcare system, it would be best to start from the beginning. Believe me, it has always been a fight. Our story might be familiar to many other Canadian families trying to navigate the healthcare system with their children. Why does it have to be this way?

THREE

THE BEGINNING

Morgan was born on a bright snowy day in February 1995, in Toronto, Ontario. She was what is referred to as a "Rainbow Baby" which essentially means that she was a healthy baby born after the loss of another baby.

Despite this heartbreaking loss and the difficulties with this pregnancy, Morgan joined our family and we were so happy.

Morgan was such an awesome baby. Yes, I know that many people say this about their babies, but she seriously was. I had 18 nieces and nephews and had quite a bit of experience with babies. Although she was my first and only child, I knew a thing or two about babies.

Morgan was so easy to please, rarely cried except for when she was hungry. She entertained herself under her Mickey Mouse jungle gym, she ate well, she slept well. Overall, it was a dream to have a baby as easy going as Morgan was.

I have this fond memory of an early morning in April 1995. It was about 2 a.m. and Morgan woke up. Scott was sound asleep. Morgan rarely woke up in the evening, so I took the opportunity to really appreciate the moment. The moon was shining through the glass patio doors in our condo at the corner of Queens Quay and Yonge Street.

I fed and changed her and of course burped her, then I just held her. I didn't want to put her down, I held on so tightly and I told her that I was so happy to be her mom. I told her I would always be there for her. I know, it seems sappy, but a moment in time that I have never forgotten all these years later, a moment I treasure.

Summertime was here and it was such a beautiful time to have a baby walking up and down the waterfront and stopping in on Scott at Queens Quay Terminal where he had a little shop set up.

On Scott's days off, we would cross the street from our condo complex, take the ferry and head out to Center Island. Center Island is a beautiful place, minutes from downtown Toronto, yet a world apart, a place where people go to forget about all the concrete and to enjoy relaxing in nature surrounded by Lake Ontario.

We relaxed and talked about where and when to get Morgan baptised. Scott being raised in the catholic faith felt that Morgan should be baptized catholic. While I was a church going protestant while growing up, I had no real feeling either way. I felt that if her father was catholic and he wanted his daughter to be catholic, so be it.

While Scott was working the following day, I contacted a nearby catholic church. I was amazed that I was speaking with a priest immediately. He introduced himself and I introduced myself and explained that we would like our daughter to be baptized in his church.

He asked me if Scott and I had been married in the church and I explained that we had not, that we made the decision to get married by the justice of the peace at Old City Hall in downtown Toronto.

I explained that Scott was catholic and really wanted his daughter baptized. The priest seemed to be upset and said that if it was our desire to baptize our daughter in the catholic faith that we should have thought about that when we got married and before she was born. He didn't miss a beat; I couldn't get a word in edgewise.

I could have continued the conversation and let him know why we decided to elope and not let anyone know. I could have told him that my mom was terminally ill and I didn't want to stress her out with a wedding. I could have told him many other things, but I realized there was no point. I needed to move on.

I told Scott about my conversation with the priest, and we agreed that Morgan would be christened by the minister that had christened me. We were excited about it, as Reverend Baugh was now at the United Church in Ste Adele, Quebec. We were looking forward to our first family trip there and then a phone call put everything on hold.

It was July 1995, Scott's Dad called from Calgary. He called often, but this was very different. As soon as Scott hung up, he told me that his sister Joanne was missing somewhere in Edmonton. I thought that was odd as Joanne lived with her boyfriend and two kids in Calgary. What was she doing in Edmonton?

It was hard for Scott to repeat what his father had said. His Sister was missing in Edmonton and the police were looking for her.

Scott and I were aware that Joanne was considering leaving her boyfriend, but it came as a shock that it happened so quickly and that she was moving in with a friend in Edmonton, and now she was missing.

Scott immediately called his mom, his parents had been divorced for a few years, so they were not together. He wanted to find out what his mom knew, maybe she was aware of more information than what Scott's Dad was.

Scott's Mom explained that his sister was staying with her friend in Edmonton and decided to go out with a bunch of friends. Joanne's friend happily stayed home with the children, as she had a child of her own. The friend called Scott's Mom, Alison and told her that Joanne didn't return from her night out. She didn't know what to do with the kid's as she had to work the next day.

Scott knew Joanne's friend and he gave her a call himself. The friend was in a state of shock, that much was obvious, she told Scott that it was very unusual for Joanne not to return home. She knew that Joanne was very excited to have a "night out" before starting her new life back in Edmonton, but she was confident that Joanne would have called her if she was unable to make it back to her house.

Scott immediately booked tickets for the three of us to head out to Calgary, and just like that our first family trip was to Calgary, Alberta.

Morgan was only five months old when we flew to Calgary to be with Scott's parents while they waited for Joanne's return.

Overall, Morgan was quite well behaved for most of the flight. We were on our descent when Morgan started crying and fussing. I remember telling Scott that I thought she was sick. He didn't think so, but when we landed and were at the gate, Scott picked her up and she vomited all over him. I'm sure he thought I was right at that moment.

As I think back to this time, I can only imagine the thoughts that were going through Scott's mind. He just got word prior to leaving, that the police in Edmonton found body parts in suitcases on the shores of the North Saskatchewan River and his daughter had just thrown up all over him.

Glen, Scott's Dad, met us at the airport. The stench of baby vomit on Scott's shirt was too much for him to handle and he had to change in the men's room.

Morgan had settled down, obviously she was sick to her stomach and had to get rid of whatever it was that was bothering her. I had only met Scott's Dad one other time, but I could tell that Glen was stressed.

He was meeting his granddaughter for the first time, and he couldn't really appreciate this because his oldest child Joanne was missing and the police had found suitcases with body parts in them.

We visited with Glen in his downtown Calgary Condo on 12th Avenue S.W. for a couple of hours, the phone was continuously ringing, people who were deeply concerned for Glen during this difficult time.

We headed to Scott's Mom's home, in Edgemont, which is in the Northwest area of Calgary. Alison was so relieved to see Scott. It was such an emotional time and I felt awkward as if I had been dumped into a personal situation where I did not belong.

I had only met Scott's family the one time when after we got married, and now this deeply emotional time was upon them. I felt I needed to step back and let them share this privately.

Of course, I had Morgan with me. I was focused on making sure that she did not disturb the family while they were sitting waiting to hear back from the Edmonton police. Thankfully at this time, Morgan was still very much an easy to please baby.

The next day, I stayed at Alison's place with Morgan while Scott and his mom went to Edmonton to discuss the body parts found in the suitcases. Unfortunately, the police confirmed that these body parts belonged to Joanne.

I headed back to Toronto from Calgary a week before Scott. It was a difficult time, as cell phones were not around and many of Scott's friends from out west were calling our condo to find out about what happened to Joanne.

At this time, no one knew what happened to her. She went out with friends and ended up murdered. It was hard to wrap our heads around. Scott stayed with his family an extra week as they mourned and tried to figure out how something like that could happen.

In August of 1995 we had our second family trip, and this was to Ste. Adele Quebec to have Morgan christened by the same Minister that had christened me, oh so many years before.

When we got back to our condo in Toronto, Scott and I discussed making the move to Calgary to be closer to his family. His Dad really seemed to need us there and his mom certainly would appreciate us there. She had her sisters to lean on, but Glen had no other family in Calgary at the time, as Lynn, Scott's other sister, lived in Saskatchewan.

We moved out to Calgary in early September 1995, and I started working as a Personal Investment Manager, with one of the top banks, in downtown Calgary.

True to Calgary form, there was a blizzard on my first day of work. I was not used to having blizzard like conditions in September, but obviously grew more accustomed to them.

So, on my first day of work, my first day of leaving my daughter at a local day care centre, I had to drive in a city that I wasn't familiar with to work in a massive snowstorm. I guess nothing says welcome to Calgary quite like these unexpected blizzards.

Shortly after I started back to work, Morgan developed ear infections. It seemed no sooner had she finished her antibiotics and then there would be another ear infection.

She also started head banging on soft surfaces. It seemed as if she would bang her head on the sofa out of frustration because she could not communicate. She also would head bang on plush carpeting if we told her no for any reason. I was confused by the head banging but felt a bit at ease, as she directed her anger and frustration to soft surfaces.

In November 1995, Joanne's remains were released to the family and there was a private burial service. When I returned from the funeral, I had a message from my sister that my mother was rushed to the hospital, and it didn't look good.

We knew that my mom wasn't in good health, she had emphysema from years of smoking which had taken a toll on her. I took a few days off from work and took Morgan back to the Laurentians, north of Montreal, to visit with my mom.

It would be the last visit that I had with my mom, but one that I cherish. Just seeing her smile when I put Morgan, who was now 10 months old, on her hospital bed was definitely a highlight of my visit.

My Mom was the first person to give my daughter chocolate and oh how she reveled in the knowledge that she was able to spoil my daughter in this way. On January 2, 1996, my Mom passed away and would not get to know my daughter.

So much had happened in the first year of my daughter's life. It seemed like one thing after another. Yet, it wasn't over, far from it. I wasn't prepared for the rollercoaster ride we were about to go on.

FOUR

DR. WONG

Morgan had countless ear infections between 7 and 11 months of age and underwent her first ear surgery in late January 1996.

My baby was under a year old, and she was going to be subjected to general anesthetic. Scott and I were not happy about this, but the ENT specialist said that once the tubes were put in place to drain her ears, that she would begin talking.

Yes, throughout everything that we had been through in 1995, it was apparent that Morgan did not speak. I can't say that she didn't say any words, because she actually said "Badoo" all the time. That one word, she said for everything. I knew that if she was pulling the fridge door it meant that she wanted to get a juice, oh did she love her juice. As a mother, it was instinctual, I knew what she wanted when she said "Badoo".

That morning of her first surgery was difficult for Scott and me since Morgan was not allowed to eat or drink. She was both a particularly good eater and she loved her juice. We told her that we had to go see a doctor and that after seeing the doctor we would go for breakfast. I doubted that she understood any of that, but it made us feel good.

After Scott handed Morgan off to the medical staff for her surgery, we both went into our respective washrooms and cried. To see your baby taken away for surgery is one of the most heart wrenching things you go through as a parent.

To our surprise, Morgan was perfectly fine in the afternoon, it seemed as if nothing had happened that day. As adults, there is certainly something we can learn from babies and the way that they handle obstacles in their lives.

Unfortunately, the ear infections continued. It was a vicious circle, ear infection, antibiotics, yeast infection and repeat. As parents, it was difficult to see our child suffer so much. However, Morgan had no time to feel sorry for herself. By now, my extremely calm baby was an energetic, overactive out of control toddler.

Understandably, people's ideas of what an out-of-control toddler is may differ. By the age of three, Morgan had already jumped into a washing machine that was running, had purposely rode her tricycle down a flight of stairs, jumped off of a platform of a 6-foot-high monkey bars, stacked wagons and a doll stroller on top of one another to escape into our neighbours yard.

She was also great at playing hide and seek at inappropriate times. One time, she hid behind the laundry room door and the only reason I found her is that I slammed the door on her finger. I had to rush her to the hospital for stitches and to tend to her broken finger.

Around 18 months of age, I took Morgan to see her Paediatrician and he asked me how many words she knew. I had to think quite hard, as she did not know any words with consistency.

She had, at times, used such words as baba for bottle or papa for grandfather and a few others, but she did not use any of these words on a regular basis. She was still using the "Badoo" word which meant everything.

I could see the concern in the doctor's face, and he told me that by now she should be using some words with consistency. I asked him if he thought it could be her ears. I asked him what he thought the issue could be. I again mentioned to him about the head banging and the fact that she only crawled at 11 months of age and walked at 15 months.

The doctor turned to me and said, "don't worry we are aware of it!". I felt that his attitude was quite condescending and for the life of me, I didn't understand how "being aware of it" was going to help. I wanted to ask, "how many years of medical school did it take you to come up with that sage advice?"

I wanted to understand why my daughter could not talk. I wanted to understand why she banged her head. I wanted to understand if any of this had to do with her delay in crawling or walking. All he would say was "don't worry about it!"

This infuriated me, how do you tell a mother not to worry about it? When you yourself said that she should be using words with consistency, and she isn't.

Why couldn't he hear the overwhelming desperation in a mother's voice. Tell me what I can do to help my child?

Due to Morgan's constant ear infections, I visited with the paediatrician a number of times over the next few months and each time he would ask me how many words she knew and each time I would tell him that she didn't have any words, she didn't say anything except "Badoo". Again, the pacifying "Don't worry about it!" were the only words he would say.

I tried in vain to get him to answer more questions. Why is she still having so many ear infections? Why isn't she speaking? Why is she banging her head and his only reply was "we are aware of it."

I tried not to worry about things, the constant ear infections, the lack of speech, the head banging, delay in crawling and walking, but it was weighing on me.

It was a heavy load. So many things were running through my mind, what could be wrong with my child? I felt so isolated, so far away from my family. I had to quit work as day care would not keep Morgan there when she was running a slight fever. Of course, with all the ear infections, I had to leave work to pick her up too many times.

I never thought that I would be a stay-at-home Mom. I mean, I could understand staying at home if you have 2 or more children, but I only had one. It seriously did not make sense.

What choice did I have, none, absolutely none! I didn't have any family in Calgary and Scott's Mom and Dad both worked.

I worked very hard to earn my CFP designation (Certified Financial Planner), and if I did not continue to work in the industry, I would lose the designation.

It was an easy decision, my daughter or three little letters. Goodbye CFP.

In late January 1997 I happened to walk past an office in Beddington Heights that said Dr. Bryon Wong, Pediatrician, accepting new patients. It was as if it was a sign from above telling me to have Morgan checked out by a different doctor.

I spoke with the receptionist, and she told me that Dr. Wong was particularly good with children. I booked an appointment for a few days later and felt as if I had renewed hope. I had to keep being positive and do whatever it took to help my daughter.

When I met with Dr. Wong, my immediate thought was that he was too young and too inexperienced. However, I quickly reminded myself about Morgan's paediatrician who was an older gentleman and had a wealth of knowledge and experience. I kept hoping that a younger doctor would have new ideas, maybe, just maybe, Dr. Wong could help us out.

Morgan occupied herself with the basket of toys in Dr. Wong's office while I spoke to him, shockingly it appeared as if he were listening, truly listening. I told him about the constant ear infections.

I rambled on and told him everything, yes everything. I told him that Morgan was the most awesome and quiet baby and just like that became an overactive out-of-control toddler.

I told him that she could not speak except for the word "Badoo " which meant everything. I did explain that she seemed to know a word for a day or so and then just like that it disappeared.

I told him how she crawled at 11 months of age and only started walking at 15 months. I didn't hold back anything. I told him of her antics, and he listened, he really listened. Before I took a breath and gave him a chance to reply, I firmly told him "Don't tell me not to worry about it!" I needed to make sure I never heard those words again.

He didn't say anything at first. He told me he would interact with Morgan and check her ears, because obviously she had another ear infection.

He played with Morgan on the floor. Yes, this doctor was on the floor with my toddler. He picked her up to put her on the examination table and she didn't complain. He checked her ears and then put her back down on the floor so that she could play with the toys in his office.

Once Morgan was busy with the toys, he said that indeed she did have an ear infection, but he was a bit concerned about her. He said, "I think that your daughter may be autistic, and I want to book an appointment for you and her to meet with the Developmental Clinic."

As we left Dr. Wong's office, so many thoughts were swirling in my mind. First off, who is this young doctor and what does he truly know? It was one appointment. I had this inner struggle because the older paediatrician said not to worry, now Dr. Wong made me worry. Isn't that what I wanted? I purposely told him not to tell me not to worry.

Again, as the internet was in its infancy, I had to rely on books. I took Morgan for an ice cream and to play in the park, as she had to have some physical activity if I expected her to go into a bookstore.

I found some books about autism and read as much as I could to try and help me understand more about it.

I was sure that we would get to the bottom of whatever issues she had. We would address them head on and with Dr. Wong's help and the help of the Developmental Clinic, Morgan would succeed and she would talk.

I decided right there and then that Dr. Wong was the pediatrician for Morgan, he was a no-nonsense doctor who wanted to help us. I don't regret this decision for a moment.

February 1997 was upon us and Morgan was scheduled for her second set of tubes. I'm once again reassured by her ENT specialist that this will help her pick up speech. She was two years old by now and still did not speak. Again, she would seem to know a word or two and then those words were gone, totally gone.

This was a very difficult surgery for me mainly because Scott had just started a new job and was scheduled for in field training and there was no way that he would be able to get out of it. Glen worked full time. Alison was working that day and Lynn was now attending the University of Calgary. It definitely would have been nice to have some of my family living closer, but I didn't and had to face the surgery on my own.

This time I drove the long drive to the hospital on my own. I had to hand off my daughter to the medical team and rush to the bathroom to cry, on my own, all of which I did.

I sat in the cold, dimly lit waiting area of the hospital, feeling so alone, wanting so much to have some family with me. I was on my own, just me and my tears. I kept reassuring myself that Morgan was soon going to be able to talk after these tubes. I kept telling myself that this was the only problem with my daughter. I kept thinking that Dr. Wong was well meaning, but my daughter has horrible ears and once these tubes were in place, she would be fine.

Once again, Morgan emerged from the surgery as if nothing happened. What incredible resilience children have! I was over the moon happy to have my daughter back. I was happy to head home with her and play with her plastic puppies that she so enjoyed.

Since our first visit with Dr. Wong, we visited him a few times and he recommended that I contact a publicly funded speech therapist.

I contacted this speech therapist before Morgan's second set of tubes and explained the situation, that Morgan's only word was "Badoo" and that she seemed to pick up a word and then totally forget it, almost as if she had never said it before. She asked me on the phone if we spoke more than one language at home and I told her that we did not. She asked if either Scott or I spoke another language and I told her that I spoke French, as I had grown up in a rural community in Quebec where French was the main language.

I really had no understanding as to why that mattered. I already clearly told her that we only spoke English at home. For whatever reason, she felt this was relevant. She said that when a child is delayed with their language skills that it could be because there are two or more languages spoken at home and that this somehow confuses children.

I was not going to argue with this woman, but many of my nieces and nephews spoke English and French at Morgan's age and my daughter was still struggling to speak one language.

She wasn't really listening to what I was saying. I had been dealing with a lot of people who really didn't listen, and it was starting to get frustrating.

FIVE

THE PAPER TICKERS

Morgan was just about three years old by the time our appointment with the developmental clinic was scheduled.

By this time, Morgan was speaking as if she had spoken at birth. There was no baby talk, no gibberish at all, Morgan was truly speaking. Both Scott and I were overwhelmed with the fact that Morgan could now speak. If you had met Morgan at three years old and I had told you of her problems with picking up speech, you never would have believed me.

Was it due to the second set of tubes? Was it due to the lessons that I learnt from the speech therapist? We knew that it wasn't from watching TV shows, as Morgan was unable to sit and watch a full half hour of T.V.

Now Dr. Wong's words seemed so far away, Morgan was coming along, and I couldn't be happier.

As I entered the developmental clinic, I was greeted by a receptionist that said a doctor would be with me shortly. I was quite impressed, we met with various therapists, including a speech language therapist, an occupational therapist, a physical therapist and various doctors and lastly the head psychologist at the clinic.

Morgan was having the time of her life. These were all new experiences to her, all the balls, all the people playing with her, she enjoyed herself immensely. She loved all the attention. I was excited to speak with the psychologist. I wanted to hear her say that Morgan was not autistic.

The psychologist said that there was absolutely nothing wrong with Morgan. She was impressed with how her speech had picked up and her overall development.

She did warn me however, that Morgan was an overactive preschooler. Believe me, I didn't need anyone to tell me this. Scott and I were both exhausted dealing with her antics. We were so excited to learn that developmentally Morgan had reached all the milestones.

By late August of 1998, Scott and I were still extremely happy with the way Morgan was speaking and that she was progressing very well. Mostly, we were happy that Dr. Wong was wrong. Although the ear infections persisted.

We both felt that Morgan, being an only child, would benefit from play school. Scott and I passionately believed that as parents we can teach her some things, but she needed to learn other things from children. Certainly, some of the things that children learn from each other are positive while others not so much.

Play school opened a whole new world for Morgan. She went twice a week for an hour and a half each time. Selfishly, I so enjoyed the 3 hours a week where I could just sit and do nothing and not worry where she was or what she was up to.

Sometimes, I would use this time to clean up the house, but most times, I did absolutely nothing and wasn't ashamed of it.

Morgan would talk incessantly about all her new friends at play school. She so loved her two teachers and absolutely loved going to play school. Ear infections aside, this was such a happy time for us as a family.

One day, towards the end of Morgan's first year at play school one of the teachers asked if she could speak with me, once all the children had left.

As I waited for all the parents to pick up their children, millions of reasons as to why the play schoolteacher wanted to speak with me went through my mind. Was Morgan not behaving in school? Was Morgan not being friendly with the other children? Was Morgan throwing tantrums? I knew she was very capable of doing so at home.

I certainly did not get this impression from Morgan. Morgan only talked positively about her whole experience, in fact she wanted to go to play school every day, instead of the two days a week.

Now it was me and the teacher, one on one, the other teacher occupied Morgan. She asked me if I ever noticed that Morgan's gross motor skills were behind. I had never heard of the term gross motor skills in my life, my background was in finance and banking, what the hell were gross motor skills?

I have since learned that gross motor skills involve movements of the large muscles of the arms, legs, and torso. Activities such as climbing, jumping, and playing in general are all done using gross motor skills.

She continued to say that when they played ball in the gymnasium both her and the other teacher noticed that there was a distinct difference in the ability of the other children to bounce a ball versus Morgan's ability.

Upon reflection, Morgan did seem awkward or clumsy. When you only have one child it's difficult to know what a child can do at a certain age versus other children. We had no one to compare her to.

After that initial shock, the teacher continued to say that they also noticed that Morgan seemed behind in her fine motor skills. Great, two new terms in one day. I knew another trip to the bookstore was in my future.

I again explained that I had no knowledge of what she meant. She explained that these were more delicate things, like holding a pencil or crayon, or using scissors. I saw that Morgan had difficulty with a pencil and with scissors but assumed that the issues were due to the fact that she was left-handed. Scott and I are both right-handed.

Since this initial introduction to the term, I have learned that fine motor skills are the coordination of small muscles and usually involves the synchronisation of hands and fingers with the eyes.

I was in complete and utter shock. Less than a year ago we were at the developmental clinic, we spent more than 4 hours there and I was told that Morgan was not delayed in any area.

I could not wrap this whole gross motor skill / fine motor skill terminology around my head. I do know that Morgan had been assessed by physical therapists and occupational therapists. Shouldn't they have pointed out these delays to me?

Why was I told that there was nothing of concern about my daughter developmentally?

Yet here the teacher is saying that in fact she does have these motor skill issues. In fact, the teacher used the term "distinct difference" between Morgan's gross motor skills and fine motor skills compared to the other children.

Even before I had a chance to speak with Scott about what the play schoolteacher had told me, I phoned Dr. Wong's office and booked an appointment to meet with him.

Everyone at Dr. Wong's office was so amazing. They were so understanding and seemed so caring of Morgan and me. When I called, and I called often, they would make sure that I got in to see him at the very latest, the same week.

I was on the verge of tears as I explained to Dr. Wong what the play schoolteacher had told me earlier that week. He reassured me that Morgan would qualify and greatly benefit from a preschool program held at the developmental clinic.

He submitted another request for Morgan to be seen and evaluated by the developmental clinic. He did tell me however, that there could be another long delay.

Morgan was already four years old. We didn't have much time before school started. I urgently wanted her to be part of the preschool program so that she would be ready to start school with the other children.

I contacted the developmental clinic and told them that I would be ready in a moment's notice if there were any cancellations.

About a month later, to my surprise, I got a call in the morning saying that there was a cancellation for the afternoon, and they would be happy to have Morgan fill it. I immediately said that I would be there, and I got Morgan ready for the appointment.

I knew that in order for Morgan to be able to focus, I would have to take her to the park, her favourite place in the world. I would have to make sure she ran a lot and burnt off energy before the appointment.

On our way to the clinic, I told her that once we were finished with that appointment we would once again spend lots of time at the park.

During my second visit to the developmental clinic, with a little experience under my belt, I approached the reception desk to let them know that we had arrived.

I did explain that I was grateful for her to arrange for Morgan to be seen so quickly. She swirled around in her chair and rudely said to me "**I don't know why Dr. Wong keeps sending you here, there is nothing wrong with your child!**"

The expression of anger surprised me, we were in a place where children and families should feel safe and comfortable. I didn't want to be combative with her, but I wanted to say "what the hell do you think would make a paediatrician refer a small child to the developmental clinic for a second time?"

Instead, I politely thanked her, and said that I honestly thought, after speaking with Dr. Wong, that Morgan would benefit from the preschool program.

I took Morgan back to the waiting area where I sat down, and she made a mad dash to the toys. She loved going to new places to discover different toys.

I tried to shake off what the receptionist told me, for the good of my daughter. I felt as if I had to gravel to get Morgan the help she needed. While I didn't appreciate it, I knew I had to do what I had to do for Morgan's benefit. After sitting in the waiting area for what seemed like an eternity, Morgan's assessment started.

In walks a young lady who introduces herself as an occupational therapist. By now, I have had enough time to learn that an occupational therapist helps people with their fine motor skills.

Morgan did not appreciate that her play time was disturbed, but I managed to coax her into an office where the occupational therapist had put things together for Morgan to do.

She had building blocks and she asked Morgan to stack the blocks. I know that the occupational therapist was not overly excited that Morgan had no patience to stack the blocks, she certainly could stack blocks, but that was not what she had wanted to be doing at that moment.

The occupational therapist continued encouraging Morgan to complete other tasks, such as colouring, again Morgan had little to no interest in colouring, and this was an area that she was weak in.

Then she asked Morgan to cut out a picture of a beach ball. Morgan loved the brightly coloured paper that was used but she tried for all of 10 seconds to cut the paper and then threw the scissors on the ground.

The occupational therapist was cordial about Morgan's frustrations, but she kept ticking off boxes on her paper. I tried to elicit some type of conversation with the occupational therapist, but she watched Morgan get utterly discouraged with the tasks that were asked of her and she just kept ticking away.

She then said that a physical therapist would be with us shortly. We waited again in the same waiting room and Morgan enjoyed returning to the toy pile. I kept thinking to myself, wondering what the occupational therapist had accomplished with all the tick marks? What was she ticking? What did this mean? Why wouldn't she talk to me since I knew Morgan better than anyone. It didn't make a lot of sense to me.

The wait this time wasn't too long and then another young lady introduced herself and took Morgan and me to a gymnasium with brightly coloured mats on the floor. Morgan's eyes lit up as she entered the room. She was familiar with these yellow, red, blue and green mats from the gym area in her play school.

The physical therapist threw a large ball to Morgan ever so delicately and Morgan caught the ball. The physical therapist asked Morgan to jump up and down and Morgan was having a wonderful time with this. She stopped from time to time to tick off some boxes. I could see the paper that she was using had boxes beside them and she was feverishly ticking those boxes. Were all these ticks good or bad, I had no idea. It was nice to see Morgan enjoying herself, especially since I knew she did not enjoy her time with the occupational therapist. The last item on the agenda was more jumping, but this was not just jumping in place, no, this was jumping from different heights.

She had Morgan jump from something that was about a foot or so off the ground, then something that was two feet or so off the ground, then she wanted Morgan to jump off from a countertop.

I wasn't comfortable with this, so I asked her if it was necessary. Morgan loved to jump off of things and I really didn't want to encourage this type of behaviour.

Morgan occasionally mentioned that she would like to climb to the roof of the garage and jump from there. I had understandable concerns, but the physical therapist did not. She insisted that it was necessary to complete her assessment of Morgan.

I was pretty sure she wrote that the child's mother was overprotective. I didn't care because she didn't live with Morgan. I did and I knew her antics.

Morgan successfully completed the jump and just like that our time with the physical therapist was over.

We returned to the same waiting room and Morgan went back to the pile of toys. So much was running through my mind. The main thing of course was wondering why anyone would want a preschooler to jump from such a high level.

I tried not to worry. I had confidence in Dr. Wong, and he told me that Morgan would greatly benefit from this preschool program. I kept telling myself that I should be thankful that we were able to be seen so quickly.

The child development specialist met us in the waiting area and brought us back to a quiet room. She asked Morgan if she liked books. Morgan was thrilled, she loved to have us read books to her.

It was a ritual of ours to read her two books every night. It was a routine we all were fond of. Morgan would pick out the two books that she wanted us to read to her and she would often sneak in a third book for us to read.

She enjoyed reading so much. With her speech delay, we were in the habit of reading books every chance we got.

Morgan definitely had a good work out with the physical therapist and was now enjoying listening to the child development specialist read a story to her. Every once in a while, the specialist would ask Morgan a question about the story that she was reading to her and Morgan replied without hesitating.

We had never read stories to her in that way. We just read stories, made silly faces, or mimicked an animal sound somewhere in the story, but we never questioned her about the stories. I thought that this was something I would want to incorporate in my daily routine with Morgan.

Once done, she said that the three specialists would discuss their findings about Morgan. She asked that I return to the area in about half an hour. I took this time to bring Morgan outside so that she could run around and be free. After the outside time, we enjoyed a treat in the cafeteria.

Morgan and I returned to the clinic area and met with the three specialists/therapists and nervously waited to hear what they had to say. Since none of them gave me any feedback while Morgan was trying to complete the tasks, they simply ticked boxes on their respective sheets of paper.

The child development specialist began by saying that the program that Dr. Wong wanted Morgan to be part of required that she be seriously behind in two of the three areas that were tested today. This was nothing new, as Dr. Wong had told me that Morgan needed to be behind in at least two areas.

My mind was swirling, I knew just from speaking with the play schoolteacher that both her fine and gross motor skills were seriously delayed.

The specialist said that it was obvious that Morgan's fine motor skills were quite delayed, but that her gross motor skills were at least two years ahead of where the average 4-year-old would be.

She continued to say that she felt that Morgan's language/comprehension skills were also advanced for her age. Therefore, according to them, Morgan was only behind in one area, she did not qualify for the program.

This was the only time that I was actually hearing from them and actually permitted to speak, so I let them know what the play schoolteacher had told me. I mentioned that there was something with the way Morgan walked that concerned the teacher as well.

I was wasting my time if I thought for one moment that anything I said would make a difference, I was only fooling myself.

According to the ticks on their pages, Morgan did not qualify. I thought back to what Dr. Wong had told me about the program and how he thought Morgan would benefit from it and that it would help her in starting school. I thought back to the conversations with the play schoolteacher and wondered why I was getting different versions of the issues Morgan had?

The main question in my head at this time was why wasn't anyone listening to me? Wasn't what I had to say important in any evaluation of Morgan?

By this time, Morgan was tired of being cooped up, she needed to get out and play and I knew this, they knew this and could see her impatience and inability to sit still for too long yet, she did not qualify.

Those words stung, I found them so hard to digest, especially since they came from three young women, who probably just graduated from university. They really did not seem to have any insight into what it was like to have a child that would greatly benefit from involvement in this program Dr. Wong spoke so highly of.

As I stood there with the paper tickers as I now called them, a lot of questions came to mind. What did they know? How could they arrive at this conclusion after they spent such little time with her? Why didn't they ask me anything? They just kept ticking the boxes!

I assumed one of the reasons that they kept the child in the room while they dismissively shared their conclusions was so that parents don't explode. I mean seriously, what could I say with Morgan being there, particularly with her screaming at the top of her lungs that she wanted to leave.

There was so much more I wanted to tell these ladies. I wanted them to know that as a mom, I desperately wanted assistance to help my daughter succeed in life.

I wanted my daughter to be able to do the things that every child does. I was in shock, serious shock, how could these paper tickers even consider that my daughter was 2 years ahead of other children when it comes to gross motor skills when that simply wasn't true.

I think that just because Morgan was not afraid to jump from a countertop that they thought she was advanced.

Such bullshit, but what could I do, the ticks were made, and Morgan was not going to be part of the program.

SIX

IS ANYBODY LISTENING?

After the evaluation, I had a follow up appointment with Dr. Wong. I described the lack of communication in the assessments, the paper ticking, and the fact that they didn't want me to explain Morgan's experiences at home or at play school. Dr. Wong was as disappointed as I was, but I knew he didn't want to show too much of his disappointment as he didn't want to discourage me.

Dr. Wong, simply being Dr. Wong listened to me, he let me speak even though the young paper tickers in the developmental clinic did not. I told him that I thought I was responsible for Morgan not being allowed into the clinic. I continued to say that I had felt that because I focused so much on her speech, language, and communication skills, because of her delay, that she had done particularly well in these areas.

Perhaps, if I had not worked so much to help Morgan, she would have been accepted into this program. I knew by the look on Dr. Wong's face that he agreed, but there was nothing either one of us could do about it.

I looked into the cost of private occupational therapy, as I felt that this was the area that we needed to focus on the most, to prepare Morgan for school.

I could not believe how expensive it was. We had decided that someone needed to stay home with Morgan to continue working with her every day to prepare her for school and essentially for life. Now only Scott was working and with only one pay cheque coming in, private occupational therapy was expensive.

After my investigation into the costs, I contacted Scott's insurance provider through his employment. I discussed with this lovely lady the issues we were facing and how Morgan desperately needed occupational therapy.

She was very pleasant and seemed to want to help but stated that normally if occupational therapy is covered it's due to an individual having had an accident or brain trauma of some sort. She said the reason that it is not covered through the employee's plan is that it is covered by public health services.

I explained to her that my daughter needed occupational therapy, but it was not covered by the public system and her issues were not due to an accident.

I pondered the situation for a day or so and then instinctively said that I needed to contact my MLA. (Member of Legislative Assembly) The MLA in my area of Huntington Hills was also the Minister of Health, how perfect could that be.

I called my MLA's office weekly and left messages with his Calgary assistant each time, finally after a few months, his assistant called me back to say that the MLA would see us.

We booked an appointment for the following week. By now, we were already working with a private occupational therapist. Our hope was that the MLA, since he was also the health minister, would understand our predicament and ensure that the developmental clinic would accept Morgan into the preschool program.

I dressed Morgan in a purple and white flowing Minnie Mouse top with the matching shorts, even had the white socks and purple running shoes. Her hair was put up into two ponytails with purple ribbons. We were ready to meet with the MLA.

The assistant said that she would occupy Morgan while I went in to speak with the MLA. I walked into his office and was surprised to see how lavish and elaborate it looked. Nice to see our tax dollars go to good use.

The MLA certainly liked to hear himself talk. He went on and on about how health care must be kept for the most vulnerable of our society first and foremost. I looked him straight in the eye and I told him that I believed a 4-year-old child is one of the most vulnerable in our society.

He was shocked at my knowledge, I had done my research, I was prepared to meet with him. I had statistics. I knew what I was talking about.

I explained how intelligent Morgan was and how she would benefit greatly by attending this preschool program. I needed to tell him our story. I wanted him to empathize with our situation and tell me that he was going to do everything he could to help.

He was so good at trying to get you to forget what you were talking about. He nodded his head, waiting for the slightest opening so he could talk. He was excellent at trying to get me to listen to him run off on a tangent.

Not this time buddy, I am going to talk, and you are going to listen. I explained that I had done a significant amount of research, keeping in mind that the internet was still in its infancy.

I told him that it was critical for children like Morgan to get assistance as early as possible to ensure their success in school and in life.

All the time and effort that I put into preparing for the meeting was a colossal waste of time. I realized this within the first five minutes. It was obvious that he didn't really care and probably tuned me out the entire time.

I was in his office for a maximum of 15 minutes, and he ended the meeting with the same line that he used when he greeted me. "Health care has to be kept for the most vulnerable of our society first and foremost."

Those were empty words. He was merely placating me. He had zero interest in listening to anything I said and even less interest in doing anything to help us.

The MLA escorted me into the main area of the office where his assistant was busy occupying Morgan. He looked at Morgan and exclaimed, "What a gorgeous little girl you are!" and just like that we left.

A few weeks later, I received a letter in the mail from my MLA thanking me for the meeting and again exclaiming how healthcare is first and foremost for the most vulnerable of our society. I tore up that letter and threw it in the garbage.

What else could a mother do? I desperately wanted to get her whatever help she needed and assumed that our healthcare system would be by our side.

We hired a private occupational therapist who came once a month. I listened and watched and made sure Morgan worked on all the tasks that the occupational therapist had shown us.

Certainly, most preschoolers enjoy beading, and play doh, but in our family this took on a whole new meaning.

Every day, and I seriously mean every day, Morgan and I took on a new beading project. When we weren't beading necklaces or bracelets, it was something related to the upcoming holiday. At Christmas, Easter, Halloween, Valentine's Day no matter what the occasion, we were beading.

As with beading, every single day we were playing with play doh and we created whatever Morgan was in the mood to create that day.

Sometimes we would be making dinosaurs, she was so fascinated by dinosaurs. Of course, it was hard for anyone else to recognize what her masterpieces were. But that didn't matter as long as her fingers were moving, I didn't care.

Unfortunately, mastering the use of scissors was not an easy task and Morgan's patience level with cutting things was non-existent.

I couldn't count the number of times that the scissors flew across the room. She really tried, and I really worked hard with her. I know that her fine motor skills were behind, but I think being left-handed in a right-handed world didn't help her.

The occupational therapist that we hired had told us to do as much finger painting as possible. She said that kids love the tactile sensation of having the wet paint on their fingers, and in this way, it would force Morgan to keep using/exercising her fingers.

Believe me, getting prepared for a finger-painting episode was a job in itself. I covered the entire table with newspaper as well as the floor beneath Morgan's chair. I knew that it was always a messy affair, but Morgan enjoyed it and it kept her fingers moving.

I had just prepared the table and floor when the phone rang. The phone was in the other room, so I went to answer it. I was on the phone for a total of three minutes.

When I came back into the kitchen, I couldn't believe my eyes. In the three-minutes that I was away, Morgan had stripped naked and painted her entire body and face along with the kitchen chairs and walls.

That ended our finger-painting pre-maturely that day as I had to give Morgan a bath and clean the entire kitchen.

The ear infections continued and as usual it was ear infection, antibiotics and then yeast infection and so on and so on. A few more surgeries to replace the ear tubes.

Morgan loved her second year of play school. This time it was three days a week for three hours each day.

This meant nine hours a week where I didn't have to worry about occupying Morgan with tasks for her fine motor skills. Nine hours a week to myself.

Sometimes, I did manage to get some work done at home. I researched how to further help Morgan with her fine and gross motor skills. To be honest, there were plenty of times where I did absolutely nothing and enjoyed every minute of it.

The summer before kindergarten, Morgan had a nine year old friend from down the street who would stop by on occasion to play with her.

I always had excellent treats out for her and Morgan. It was a relief to have someone other than myself occupy Morgan.

I was in the kitchen when the friend came bursting into the house from the garage where they had been playing. She was screaming saying that Morgan had jumped off the roof of the car onto the cement padding of the garage floor.

I had trouble processing what she was saying because she was so frantic. I just ran out to the garage and sure enough Morgan was getting up from the garage floor and I could see the blood oozing from her forehead.

I am not sure if I contacted this young girl's mother to come pick her up or if she walked home by herself, she only lived about six houses down the street.

Morgan and I were off to the hospital again. My heart was pounding, I told Morgan to keep the wet cloth on her forehead while I drove to the emergency room.

Scott was out of town on business once again, and I was there with Morgan on my own. I didn't want to call him until I had more information from the hospital. I kept hoping I was panicking for nothing.

No, it was not nothing, Morgan required stitches, dissolvable ones that would not leave a mark, the doctor said. She was such a trooper, I sat with her while they froze her forehead and then did the stitches.

I don't know if it was for her benefit or my own, but I told her that if she cooperated with the doctors while they were fixing her forehead that we would go to McDonald's afterwards.

I was so happy to hear that the stitches would not leave a mark on her forehead but was not so excited to hear that I would have to watch over her for signs of a concussion.

I was on my own with Morgan that night, plenty of time to think about how nice it would be to have some family close by to lean on during tough times, but I didn't have any so that was that.

I was not the type of person to dwell on the negative, I allowed myself a few moments of self-pity and carried on.

I didn't sleep a wink that night as I watched over my daughter for signs of a concussion. Now that the trauma of the event had somewhat subsided, I thought back to the appointment we had had at the developmental clinic where the physical therapist had asked Morgan to jump from the counter. Could this have given Morgan a false sense that if she jumped from the car roof, she wouldn't hurt herself?

Thankfully, Morgan didn't have a concussion and the next day when she got up, she was not one bit concerned about her forehead or the stitches. Her strength amazed me.

SEVEN

WHERE'S MORGAN

Kindergarten was upon us. I was excited for Morgan because I believed that she would grow and learn so much in kindergarten.

I was happy to know that she would get the opportunity to meet other children in the Huntington Hills area. I thought back to my childhood and how I went to school with the same children that lived near me in my small town in Quebec. I so enjoyed going to school and playing with Debbie, Susan and Doris and then being able to play with them after school. I was hoping that Morgan would have a similar experience.

Morgan's kindergarten was in the morning, so she had the afternoons off. Yes, as excited as I was for Morgan to learn and grow in kindergarten, I was equally happy to have this time off.

At this point though, the time off was less for me and more for preparing things for Morgan. I planned activities that would help her with both her fine and gross motor skills.

In essence while she was in school, I researched and prepared for what we would be doing in the afternoon when she returned from kindergarten. Keeping in mind that she was only five years old, I had to ensure that anything I prepared for us to do had to hold her interest.

Morgan was not a child that could sit still for too long. At this point, she could barely sit and watch a half hour T.V. show. Even her favourites, like Blue's Clues, Bear in the Big Blue House, Barney, Bananas in Pajamas and of course her favourite show, The Powerpuff Girls could not hold her attention for too long.

The Powerpuff Girls could hold her attention the most, as these young, animated girls were always up to something. They were always running, jumping, and of course screaming, Morgan liked to imitate them, sometimes she would be Blossom, other times she preferred to be Bubbles and of course she did enjoy imitating Buttercup.

I loved that they showed these young girls as strong and independent, but sometimes they seemed to be too fearless.

I imagine that for many children this might be good, to help them come out of their shell. Morgan had no fear and I wondered if these young girls encouraged this no fear attitude even further.

As happy as I was to have Morgan in kindergarten, I did worry about the class size. There were thirty-nine other children. I knew by looking at the space available that it would be a challenge for any teacher with that many rambunctious children.

There were two teachers and an assistant in her class. I wonder why they didn't separate the classes into two and make it more manageable. Despite my concerns, Morgan enjoyed kindergarten and made many friends.

Shortly after kindergarten started, Morgan got the idea of "running away". Scott and I weren't sure where this idea came from.

Was it from a movie that we had watched, and she stopped for a minute to take a look? She certainly wasn't sitting through a movie. Had something caught her attention and we weren't even aware of it?

Was it something on one of those children shows that she barely sat down long enough to watch? She certainly was a young girl with a sense of adventure, but "running away" did not seem to be a term that she had ever encountered.

One afternoon, shortly after Scott came home from work, Morgan told us that she was going to run away.

Scott and I smiled at each other as we watched our little girl pack her Barbie suitcase. She was methodical in her packing.

She packed a spoon, a yogurt cup that she had taken from the refrigerator, an apple, then she headed to her room and packed her pajamas and a sweater. We both watched Morgan as she continued her packing, it was so comical.

Morgan opened the door and announced that she was running away. Scott was right behind her. She walked down the block responsibly on the sidewalk rolling her Barbie suitcase behind her, as she walked, she would look back.

Scott thought she did this to make sure she could still see our house. He hid behind trees and bushes so that Morgan did not see him following her.

After a few minutes, Morgan began to cry. Scott was right there, he picked her up and told her not to cry. Morgan was relieved to have her dad so close and they walked home together.

We talked to her about running away. We explained the many reasons it wasn't a good idea. Was she really listening? It seemed as though she was always thinking of her next adventure. She kept us on our toes.

Unfortunately, the next time Morgan ran away she didn't announce it. It was a beautiful sunny Saturday afternoon. Scott, Morgan, and I were outside playing jump rope and introducing Morgan to what was involved in track and field.

We also spent some time playing bubbles with our German Shepherd dog, Candy. Candy loved to catch bubbles. Morgan laughed and laughed as she watched Candy. It was fun to see them bonding in this way.

Scott and I were very tired from all this running and jumping and playing with the dog, but Morgan wasn't.

Scott and I went inside for a much-needed break and Morgan stayed out in the fully fenced back yard with Candy. The dog was very protective of Morgan. I felt comfortable leaving her outside for a few minutes with the fence and the dog. There was no way she could go anywhere. Or at least that's what we thought.

Every few minutes I would check on Morgan in the backyard. I could see her running and trying to play ball with the dog.

When I looked out the next time, she was gone. How could it be? The fence is at least five feet tall. Candy was in the backyard the whole time, but she is gone.

I panicked at this point. I run into the house and tell Scott that Morgan is missing. He runs to the basement to see if she is hiding in closets or the laundry room, anywhere.

I search the main level, all the closets, in the shower, under the beds. We are frantically calling her name. We know that she's done this before.

She hides in the house and even though we call out her name, she continues to hide, she definitely took hide and seek too literally.

We rushed back outside. Scanning the whole yard, heart, and mind racing. That's when we saw how she must have done it.

She stacked her large plastic toys up against the side of the fence, we looked over into our neighbour's backyard and noticed that her gate to the back alley was open. Sure enough, this is what Morgan had done. She climbed the toys and jumped into the neighbour's yard and ran away.

Where was she? Instinct took over, Scott took his truck and started going up and down the streets in the neighbourhood, while I frantically called 911.

The 911 operator kept telling me to calm down as I tried to explain to her that Morgan was missing. She kept insisting that it was a kidnapping. This did not make me feel better. It added to my anxiety. Even though I could see how she probably got out, I was so frightened.

I was in the backyard at this point during my conversation with the 911 operator because I thought perhaps, I could see Morgan down the back alley.

By now, the neighbours heard my wails, my screaming, and the panic in my voice and knew something was wrong.

I was on the back deck, Candy was aggressively barking at my neighbour, who at this point was trying to open the back gate. I screamed over the sounds of Candy's barking and told him that Morgan was missing.

He said that he would go out and look for her. All the while this 911 operator kept insisting that she was kidnapped. Of course, this thought did enter my mind, but how could someone come into the backyard without Candy making a scene? Candy would never let anyone into the back yard, even if we were outside, she gave people a hard time if they were near our fence.

I tried to explain this, of course, I was hysterical, but I did try to get the 911 operator to understand that no one could have gotten in the yard without us knowing because of Candy.

She did her best to calm me down but let me tell you when your five-year-old child is missing, calming down is never going to happen.

I told the 911 operator that I was going to hang up so that I could go out and look for Morgan. I felt useless while Scott and now my neighbour were out looking for her. She told me not to leave the home in case Morgan came back. Someone needed to be there if she came back.

I tried not to focus on the "if" part of her statement. Morgan was going to come back, wasn't she? Where could she be? I headed out to the front yard still on the phone with 911.

More and more people were meeting me in the front yard, Candy was barking out back, but she was secure in the backyard, as more and more neighbours came by and then headed out to find her. I sat on the front steps of our small bi-level on Huntington Way feeling defeated.

I replayed the events in my mind. Scott and I had gone into the house. I checked on her every few minutes and she was happily playing with Candy and now she is gone.

I've heard many people on the news talk about leaving their child unattended for five minutes and then they were kidnapped. I kept trying not to think this way.

I was confident Candy would never let anyone into our backyard. She would have barked and barked. This made me feel a bit better. I was fairly confident she left on her own. But where was she now?

I see the large plastic toys leaning against the fence. I see my neighbours' gate to the back alley open. I know what she did. She ran away. No, my daughter was not kidnapped.

I alternated from the front yard to the back yard all the while the 911 Operator kept talking to me. By this point, I wasn't really speaking with her, I was just holding the phone.

So many neighbours came by, and I had to tell them that Morgan was missing. Besides, this 911 Operator was not making me feel good talking about "if" she comes home and that she was probably kidnapped, I had to spend my time going from front to back looking for my daughter.

Scott would drive by, and I could see that he had been crying. Each time he came by I would let him know that I had not heard anything and that she was still missing.

He searched every street, every playground that she was familiar with. We were going crazy and worst of all we couldn't be together as support for each other. He had to be out there looking for her and I had to stay home.

Where were the police? I'd been on the phone for a long time, and they still hadn't arrived. My daughter was missing, I needed the police to help find her.

I ask the 911 Operator what's taking so long? She assured me that they are on their way. They were not there, but thankfully all the wonderful neighbours on Huntington Way were there, thankfully we had an army of people out looking for her.

It must have been about a little over an hour into the ordeal when a car stopped in front of the house. I didn't recognize the car, but I looked in the back seat and there was Morgan with her Barbie suitcase.

I was shaking and screaming so much that I had a hard time opening the back door of the car to get Morgan. My arms felt weak. I had trouble picking her up from the back seat.

I looked at her and she seemed puzzled as to why all the commotion. Why was I in tears and why were so many neighbours hanging around?

I told the 911 operator that I no longer needed the police, that some good people had brought Morgan back home to me. The wonderful couple who found her, I hugged them for what seemed like an eternity.

I didn't want to let them go, perhaps because I was so weak from crying so much that I needed to lean on someone. I continued to hug them, I cried and cried and cried.

As I pulled away from her, I finally recognized who she was. She owned a small sporting goods store not too far from where we lived. She recognized Morgan and asked her where I was. Morgan told her that she had run away from home.

Scott arrived just as the wonderful people left. He picked up Morgan and he held her so tightly and cried. Morgan was not phased at all, she seemed so confused as to why all the attention to the situation, she had just "run away".

We thanked our neighbours who had stopped whatever they were doing to look for our daughter. We were relieved and went into the house. Candy was also happy that all seemed back to normal.

Not long after we got inside, the police showed up. I was quite surprised to see them, as I had told the 911 operator that Morgan had been found. We needed them earlier to help look for Morgan. But now that she was home safely, it seemed pointless for them to stop by.

The police officers did speak with Morgan and told her that it was important to stay with Mom and Dad. Honestly, Morgan was not one bit concerned about what they were telling her, she didn't care one bit.

The police then turned to Scott and me and in a condescending tone told us that we were extremely lucky that Morgan was returned unharmed, as if we didn't already know this.

Before they left, a female officer turned to me and said, **"You watch your little girl, you know we have better things to do than look for a missing five-year-old!"**

For the life of me, I could not think of one thing more important for the police to be doing than looking for a missing child. Not one thing.

When I finally calmed down, I told Scott what the couple that found Morgan had told me. She was at a corner store on Beddington Boulevard. This would have meant that a small little girl crossed two major intersections dragging a Barbie suitcase and not one person batted an eye.

Even more concerning was the fact that Morgan had a quarter in her pocket, she told me that a man in the store gave her the quarter to buy candy.

Ok, I'm thankful that my daughter is fine, but what the hell did this man give her a quarter for?

I also wondered why the owner of the small convenience store, who had seen me in the store several times with Morgan before, had not called the police.

Even if he didn't recognize Morgan, why didn't he call the police because there was a small unaccompanied child in his store.

Over the next few days, we were terrified that Morgan might run away again, we were both quite upset about the officer's comments and thought about lodging a complaint.

How dare she talk to us like that? What could be more important than looking for a missing child. We thought about lodging a complaint, but we did not. We didn't because we were terrified that our daughter would run away again, and they would not be as enthusiastic to help us find her knowing that we had lodged a complaint.

Any parent will tell you when your child goes missing that your mind wanders to places you never thought were possible. I kept wondering what I could do to make sure this never happened again.

Surely, she learnt her lesson. Yet, I knew that she seemed undeterred from the whole experience. She was only five and didn't care about what the police officers told her.

She was just having fun and she seemed to like this thing called "running away"! While I went over and over many ways to ensure that Morgan never disappeared again, some thought was given to putting a fish net over our backyard.

This seemed weird, but it was an idea that popped into my head. Our backyard was not that big, and it would not take too much work. We could get five-foot fence posts and attach them to the existing fence, we could staple the fish net to the fence, she could not possibly escape this. After things calmed down, the fish net idea did seem totally ridiculous, and I knew I was just grasping at straws.

    I never wanted to feel that helpless again when it came to my daughter and yet I did so many more times.

EIGHT

STRAWBERRY, BLUEBERRY AND GREEN APPLE

The following week I booked an appointment with Dr. Wong while Morgan was in kindergarten. I needed to speak with him without her hearing me. I didn't want to encourage her to run away again, nor did I want her to think I was making a big deal out of the ordeal.

Dr. Wong, as always, was phenomenal. He suggested that I contact a private psychologist to see what their opinion was on how to best help Morgan. We both knew that grade one was around the corner.

I left his office feeling more positive. He had a way of giving me good advice and I really appreciated having him as a sounding board. It was obvious that he truly cared and honestly wanted to help Morgan.

I immediately called the psychologist and booked an appointment for the following week. So many questions came to mind after I had booked the appointment. Morgan had visited the developmental clinic already without any help being offered, what would the difference be with visiting a private psychologist?

Why did we have to visit a private psychologist? Why hadn't the developmental clinic helped us? I thought about the excessive wait time in the public system versus the private. I thought about how many other children like Morgan were being cast aside by the public system. I didn't want to think too much about this, as it brought me down and I didn't want to let myself go there. I couldn't change the system, I had to learn to work within it. I had to do everything that I could to help Morgan succeed whether it was through the publicly funded system or the private system.

After searching for a parking lot along 14th Street N.W., we parked and headed into the psychologist's office. This woman seemed phenomenal, she greeted Morgan first, and made her feel important.

She wanted to show Morgan that her focus was on her. After my experience with the developmental clinic, it was purely amazing meeting this woman. I immediately felt a sense of relief.

Unfortunately, it happened to be a gorgeous day outside and Morgan did not want to sit and talk with the psychologist, nor did she want to play any of the games that she had initiated. Not only was this embarrassing, but I couldn't help but think of the fact that we were paying this woman by the hour.

The psychologist recommended that I take Morgan out to the park down the street. Right there and then, I knew that this woman had experience in dealing with children.

Morgan needed to run and jump and play before she was able to sit down and concentrate on any of the activities asked of her. The sun was nice and bright as Morgan climbed the monkey bars. Oh, how she loved to climb.

I pushed her on the swing set but wanted her to be even more physical. I encouraged her to run around the playground yard. I would chase her just to get her to keep running.

We headed back to the psychologist's office and Morgan seemed more prepared to work with her now. As I sat in the waiting area listening to Morgan, I was utterly amazed at some of her responses to the psychologist.

Morgan seemed mature for her age. She was just 5 years old but had so much wisdom. Morgan was with the psychologist for about half an hour when the door opened. The psychologist asked me if I would take Morgan back out to the park again.

Morgan and I went to the park at least twice a day on average, this is something that she thoroughly enjoyed. She loved the see saw, she loved climbing the monkey bars, and in the park near our house, she particularly loved the rocking/swinging horses.

There were three horses at the park on Huntington Green and Morgan had names for them, the blue one was Blueberry, the red one was Strawberry and the Green one was Green Apple. What an imagination this child had. She had hoped that this park on 14th Street NW would have Blueberry, Strawberry and Green Apple, but unfortunately it did not.

Both of us were getting tired, it had already been a long day. Now I had to think of a way to keep Morgan busy outside in a park that did not have Blueberry, Strawberry and Green Apple. We did the usual running and climbing and swinging, then I made up a game. I was actually amazed at myself for thinking on my feet so quickly. This was not the only game that I would make up in the course of Morgan's young life. I had to be quite creative when it came to entertaining and educating Morgan.

The playground equipment was on shredded rubber so that when the children fell, they would not get hurt. There was a boarded frame built around this rubber to ensure that it did not spread all over the area.

I told Morgan to pretend that the rubber was water and we had to balance ourselves on the border and walk all around the frame. The rules implied that if your foot went off the frame you had to start all over again. Of course, this was an excellent game for her, it kept her interest and she loved acting as if she were drowning in the rubber/water when one of her feet slipped off the border. It obviously was great for her balance and coordination.

We spent about 20 minutes at the park the second time. When we returned Morgan was eager to work with the psychologist. Within a half an hour they were both out of the little office. Morgan was excited to play with the toys in the waiting area while the psychologist spoke with me.

She asked me if I had ever heard about ADHD which stands for attention deficit hyperactivity disorder. I had most certainly heard of ADHD but at that time, was under the impression that only boys had ADHD, keeping in mind that the internet was in its infancy.

Of course, the psychologist corrected me and said that there certainly were more boys than girls diagnosed with ADHD, but it was not exclusive to boys. Once again, my head was swirling, and I was trying to understand everything that she was telling me.

I was having trouble doing so, my mind was thinking back to the appointments at the developmental clinic, the discussions with child psychologists, occupational therapists, physical therapists, and child development specialists.

The private psychologist told me that there was a significant difference in what Morgan could accomplish when she returned from playing at the park.

She added that it was obvious Morgan required movement to enable her to focus. She said that she would send us a letter detailing her findings. On the drive home, I could not believe how much sense the private psychologist made.

I thought back to the second trip to the developmental clinic and how Morgan was so much better able to focus on reading with the child developmental specialist because she did so much physical work with the physical therapist.

These people are educated in child development, why didn't they point this out to me? I thought back to how pre-occupied they were in ticking off things on their paper, perhaps too busy ticking to notice or appreciate my daughter and her struggles.

About a week later, the report came in. I was nervous to open the envelope. What would it say? Would she have recommendations? Did it really matter what she said, would it make any difference in Morgan's life?

I brought the envelope to the next appointment with Dr. Wong. He reviewed everything and while he concurred with most of what the private psychologist had written, he was not as confident with the label of ADHD.

Dr. Wong felt that at 5 years of age, you could not ascertain with certainty whether a child had ADHD or not. He cautioned me by saying that he is not saying that Morgan does not have ADHD, just that at such a young age a determination could not be made.

I left there wondering why no one could seem to agree on anything when it came to my daughter. I trusted Dr. Wong, so I kept what he said front of mind and continued working with Morgan.

Every day was a commitment to working on Morgan's fine motor skills. We worked on beading, finger painting, block stacking, and cookie making. Everything was centered around making Morgan use her fingers.

So much planning and work went into everything we did to ensure that Morgan was exercising those fingers, building muscle memory so that fine motor tasks would not be so difficult for her.

I really would love to say that all our hard work was paying off. Although we were still working with a private occupational therapist and working every day on improving Morgan's fine motor skills, they were not improving.

We loved our neighbours in Huntington Hills and didn't want to leave. However, we were told that there would only be two grade one classes the following year. There were 40 children in Morgan's morning kindergarten class and another 40 in the afternoon class.

We were told that as with any school, there would be some migration and they didn't think that either class would have over 36 children in it. We knew that there would be too many children for Morgan to succeed.

I called a school close to Redwood Meadows and was informed that they only ever had 21 children in their grade 1 – 3 classes. Scott and I briefly talked about private schools as an option, but both of us were small town kids and we enjoyed hanging out with the kids that we saw in the classroom, private school was not an option we would consider. Oh, how time can change one's opinion.

So, we made the decision to move to Redwood Meadows. It was a big decision, and it wasn't made lightly. This meant that Scott would have to travel into the city via Highway 8, which is a single lane highway in both directions.

But the beauty in Redwood Meadows was limitless. The trees alone made us feel as if we could breathe. The river was quite close, and we knew right away that it was the right decision for us.

Prior to the start of grade one, I met with Dr. Wong one more time and we discussed the private psychologist's report. I wanted to know if I should bring the report to the teacher the first day so that she could be made aware of Morgan having ADHD or at least suspected of having ADHD.

As always, Dr. Wong was incredible, he was two steps ahead of the school. He said that I should not provide the school with this report, as they would judge her with it. He made a valid point that if Morgan behaved a certain way or said a certain thing or was fidgety that it was due to her ADHD. He said that it would be best to forget about the report for now and not advise the school. I thought his words of wisdom were ingenious and as a result, I did not bring the report to the school.

First day of grade one was upon us, and it was a bittersweet day for me. I was happy that Morgan was growing and would be in school full day, but I wanted my daughter to remain my little girl and I knew that grade one was the start of her becoming more and more independent.

Scott took the morning off work so that both of us could see her off to grade one. She absolutely refused to allow us to take her to school that first day. She was a "big girl" and wanted to ride the school bus like all the other children.

Scott, Morgan, and I waited at the corner for the school bus and when it came, she climbed the stairs and looked back at us and waved. I cried so much as I rushed to my car. I was going to follow the bus; I wasn't ready for her to be this grown up yet. I had to see for myself that she got to the school and wasn't upset.

I watched as Morgan got off the bus and followed the other children to the school doors. Morgan had no idea that I had followed her, and I didn't want her to know that I had done this. As Morgan walked towards the school doors, I noticed a teacher approach her and welcome her and off they went into the school.

I sat in my car and cried, I didn't want to cry, I had no idea why I was crying, but I needed to cry.

First day of grade one seemed to imply so much for children. They were no longer babies at home, they were old enough to venture out on their own without their parents. Most parents are somewhat anxious about this day, many are sad that their little ones are leaving home while others are quite happy to have their children become more independent.

I knew that Morgan had some struggles, struggles that the school were unaware of, struggles that might make it a little more difficult for her to adjust to school life than most six-year-olds.

I had to just let go of things, let things happen as they will. I had to let Morgan grow up and I knew that she so desperately wanted to grow up and be like all the other children.

The crying was perhaps a release of all my emotions, all the fighting that I had done to get Morgan to this point, perhaps it was simply the fact that my little girl was growing up and now going to school full time, perhaps it was some combination of the two.

I met Morgan at the bus stop after her first day and she was so excited about school, she was talking about her new friends and her new teacher. It was such a relief.

I was so happy that her first day went well. I was confident that she would do well in school and continue to make so much progress.

I tried to keep a positive attitude and move forward. But it always seemed like there were roadblocks everywhere we turned.

NINE

THE SHOPPING CART

The teacher liked to have parents as volunteers in the classroom. I was so happy to be a volunteer, but I wasn't very happy to discover that there were 30 children in the grade one classroom. The reason we decided to make the move out of the city was due to the fact the administration office told me that they never have more than 21 children in a classroom.

I talked with the administration and was told that this was the first year that there were so many children in grade one, but unfortunately not enough children to make two grade one classrooms.

With the volunteer schedule in place, I was in the classroom at least every other week and I got to see firsthand how the children were progressing.

I enjoyed working with all the children, and it gave me a good idea of how Morgan fared in terms of her progress. There were children that were more advanced than she was, but there were children that were more behind. Overall, I would say that she was middle of the pack.

It quickly became apparent to Morgan's first grade teacher that she was behind in her fine motor skills. The teacher was a bit older, and I felt confident with her experience and knew that Morgan was in the right class.

She explained that she was deeply knowledgeable and experienced in working with children that were behind in their fine motor skills.

Just speaking with the teacher and discovering her passion for working with children who experienced a fine motor skill delay took so much stress off my shoulders. Finally, it seemed as if Morgan was where she needed to be to succeed.

The summer in between grade one and grade two was phenomenal. Morgan enjoyed living in Redwood Meadows, she enjoyed having friends over or visiting their homes. She was a very happy little girl.

We still had to work every day on her motor skills, we continued to pay for a private occupational therapist to work with Morgan and every day we would work on both her gross and fine motor skills in fun ways.

We would take walks in the forest along the riverbanks. We played on the trampoline which we had bought to help Morgan with her balance and coordination.

Every day I had to plan what we were going to do that day that would help Morgan practice both her fine and gross motor skills. Whatever I created for her would have to keep her interest, that was for sure.

It was during these long walks that Morgan first complained of having a sore hip. She indicated to me that she could not walk from one side of the community to the other along the riverbanks.

I did find this very strange that a six-year-old would find it difficult to walk a path that I had no issue walking. Originally, I just kept thinking that perhaps she pulled a muscle with all the walking we had done that summer, or perhaps she had injured herself playing soccer with her dad. It was on my mind, and it did make me wonder, but I couldn't fixate on it.

Morgan never liked dolls, not for one minute, I have always enjoyed dolls of all kinds as a child and even as an adult.

When I was a young girl, my dolls were my world and everyone around me knew this. I had picked up some older Barbie dolls and accessories at a few different garage sales and thought that this could be a great experience for Morgan. I thought perhaps by playing with these small dolls, dressing them, putting on their shoes, that this would work Morgan's fine motor skills.

The frustration that Morgan felt trying to dress these dolls and change their shoes was quite visible as Barbies and accessories went flying across the room.

How silly of me to think that a passion of mine would become a passion of hers. No, Morgan never liked dolls and never would, especially these little ones that caused frustration to many who dare attempt to change their clothing.

However, I held out hope. At one of these garage sales there was a little sailboat for a Barbie. I knew how much Morgan loved going to the river and enjoyed being outdoors. I didn't want to give up on Barbies quite yet and so on our daily walk to the river, I brought the sailboat and a Barbie. It was a beautiful day for a sail down the Elbow River.

Morgan loved to see Barbie floating down the river, the water was so cold, but I would go in and get the boat so that Morgan could place it in the river and together we would watch Barbie float.

The wind picked up and somehow, Barbie's sailboat escaped the area that I had secured for her. She was now full on floating down the river heading towards Calgary.

Morgan looked perplexed, you could see that she did not care about the doll, but that sailboat that she so enjoyed was now drifting away. It all happened so quickly, I looked at Morgan on the banks of the river and I looked at Barbie floating away.

I felt confident that I could catch up to Barbie and complete the rescue mission. I was just about to wade further into the river when I turned back and saw Morgan. She wanted to save that sailboat and as much as I wanted to retrieve it for her.

I could not even attempt to get it. The Morgan I knew could not be trusted on the banks of the river on her own. The river was fast flowing at this point, and I knew that Barbie just had to keep floating.

This had been my chance, my last chance to have my daughter show interest in dolls and this interest was floating down the river. We waved good-bye to Barbie and wished her safe travels.

Morgan laughed off this experience. I certainly was more devastated over the loss than she was. We laughed and imagined where Barbie and her sailboat ended up. We talked about Barbie and her unplanned trip for weeks to come.

In the end, with Morgan's blessings, we ended up giving all her Barbie dolls and accessories to a friend in the community that absolutely loved everything Barbie.

Preparing for grade two, most parents get caught up in buying new shoes and new clothes and for the most part, kids love this time of year.

Morgan was never much of a shopper, and it seemed even much less so now. We headed to Chinook Mall in Calgary at the intersection of McLeod Trail and Glenmore Trail to look for a few items.

It was so embarrassing, Morgan insisted that we go to Zellers first so that we could get a shopping cart. She said that there was no way that she could walk the whole mall.

I wanted to go to Zellers last as this is where I had wanted to shop to buy her school supplies, but I had a few other stores to go to. I wanted to check a few of the children's stores to see what type of clothing was available for Morgan.

I wanted to be prepared, I wanted to make sure that any shoes she wore had velcro, as tying shoes up was still very difficult for Morgan.

I wanted her clothes to have elastic waist bands and velcro instead of buttons and zippers, things the average parent doesn't have to worry about when their child is going into grade two.

I caved in and stopped at Zeller's. Here was my 7-year-old sitting in the open area of the cart. I didn't seem to have much of a choice at that point, we had driven all the way from Redwood Meadows to get school supplies, I wasn't about to turn around.

I wondered what could be up with the fact that she couldn't walk around the mall. It was something else to worry about. It was something I would have to investigate.

We went through the mall with Morgan sitting in the basket part of the shopping cart and while we did elicit a few stares here and there for the most part, no one seemed to care.

We stopped at a few different stores. I seriously wasn't finding anything that I liked for Morgan to wear. Everything seemed to have belts, buckles, ties, ribbons, zippers and laces, all things that I was desperately trying to avoid.

Thankfully Morgan didn't really care much about what she wore, and she wasn't the type of child that would cause a scene because she wanted a certain outfit but couldn't get it. After seeing what was available in the stores, I told Morgan that we would get patterns and have her clothes made by a seamstress.

The following week we headed to the Walmart's in Westbrook Mall in Calgary on 37th Street S.W. Morgan seemed to enjoy looking at the patterns.

I explained how the pictures of the outfits were exactly what the lady (seamstress) was going to make for her. I looked for patterns that seemed to be easy for Morgan to put on and off by herself yet were fashionable.

I didn't want Morgan to stand out. I just wanted her to feel comfortable in her clothing and not to have difficulty with them. Once we picked out the patterns, we went to the material area of the store.

We picked out material that was Morgan approved, as she was quite sensitive to different textures. We headed to the seamstress where Morgan was measured. A few weeks later, we picked up the clothes and they were just gorgeous.

This seamstress did a remarkable job and Morgan loved them. She was comfortable in them, and they were easy for her to manage. Of course, these were much more expensive than store bought, but one less thing to worry about.

Grade two was quickly upon us and I started to feel slightly bored at home. Here I was a Certified Financial Planner without the credentials of a Certified Financial Planner because I had left the industry to care for Morgan.

As luck would have it the local community newspaper had a job posting for an administrative assistant to work flexible part-time hours. The posting was for a local area summer camp that catered to children with disabilities. I thought it sounded perfect.

I got the job and was so excited to be able to work only while Morgan was in school, this meant that I could drive her to school, go to work and pick her up after school.

Of course, after school we would have to work on Morgan's fine motor skills, gross motor skills, complete the grade two homework and get ready for the next day. The money was not great, but it got me out of the house, and I was so excited to be back in the workforce.

It seemed to work out perfectly until one afternoon when I went to pick Morgan up from school. Her grade two teacher, which happened to be the same teacher from grade one, indicated that she was concerned about Morgan's reading ability.

She felt that Morgan was quite behind the other children in this area. She continued to tell me that she had referred Morgan to the school's speech language pathologist as she felt that Morgan had difficulty articulating certain words. Morgan had spent some time with a speech language pathologist when she was just over two years old, but I thought that her speech was fine. She had been to the developmental clinic twice and both times no one mentioned that she had difficulty articulating any words.

I guess our journey within the healthcare system had not come to an end. I contacted Dr. Wong that same day and booked an appointment to see him.

I told him what the teacher had said. I mentioned that I thought it seemed odd that Morgan knew how to read early grade two words, but when you put them in a sentence, she couldn't read the sentence.

As an example, a simple sentence from early grade two would be something like...... The dog ran. Three simple little words. Individually, Morgan could read The and she could read dog and she could read ran but put them in a sentence and she could not read the sentence.

How could this be, what was I missing? Dr. Wong explained that it could be a visual issue and he referred Morgan to an optometrist that specializes in working with children that had visual issues pertaining to learning.

So, there I sat in the doctor's office feeling overwhelmed once again. I always recognized that people had it far worse than us, but it was still so hard to go from one issue to the next, like a never-ending story.

I just wanted Morgan to have a regular childhood. I wanted her to run and play and not have to visit one therapist after the other. I was hoping this would be the end of the issues for her. I couldn't have been more wrong.

TEN

THIRD TIMES A CHARM

We had an appointment to meet with the optometrist within a week. I couldn't help but be amazed at how much faster the private system was over the public one. The office was downtown Calgary, and the appointment time was pretty close to the lunch hour. Morgan was excited because she knew that after the appointment that we would meet up with her dad at the Keg Steakhouse on 12th Avenue SW.

The doctor was amazing and so very patient with Morgan. It was a proud moment because Morgan was so co-operative with her, yes it may come as a shock, but Morgan wasn't always co-operative with people in the medical field. Perhaps, she was as fed up as I was with the whole system.

At the end of the appointment, just when I had expected the doctor to say that Morgan needed glasses, both Scott and I wore glasses, so it was a given. No, she said that Morgan's vision was perfect.

She explained that Morgan had a visual motor skill issue. In a matter of a few years, I had become an expert on all types of motor skill issues. Or so I thought! I knew nothing about visual motor skills, but by now I was very familiar with fine motor skills and gross motor skills.

The doctor explained that visual motor skills are essential to enable us to coordinate the efficient use of our hands and eyes. Visual motor integration is a skill we require for functioning.

I tried to take all of this in, it was a bit overwhelming. The doctor continued and explained that visual motor skills enable an individual to process information around them.

She further explained that visual motor skills include a coordination of visual information that is perceived and processed with other motor skills. Visual motor skills are needed for coordinating the hands, legs, and the rest of the body's movements with what the eyes perceive.

Morgan's main issue seemed to be tracking, meaning that instead of seeing the previous sentence..... The dog ran. She saw Thedogran. She was unable to process the space between the words. So, while she was comfortable with three letter words at this point, she was not familiar with a nine-letter word, because that is what she saw, one big word instead of three little ones.

While I could not comprehend everything that she was saying, I started to understand a little bit more about Morgan and everything that she was going through, how confusing and frustrating the world must be for her. Now that I knew this, my first question was can we do anything about this?

Of course, there was vision therapy that was available. But it also meant that we would have to work a lot at home with Morgan on her vision exercises.

For anyone not familiar with vision therapy, it is important to note that it is not covered by the Alberta health care system and as far as I know is not covered by any provincial health care plan.

So, on top of paying for an occupational therapist, we would now have to pay for a vision therapist. We booked an appointment for the following week and rushed off to meet Scott for lunch.

Downtown Calgary during an oil boom meant that there was lots of hustle and bustle on the streets during lunch time and today was no different as we scurried off to meet Scott at the Keg.

Scott was sitting at a booth when we got there and the first words out of his mouth related to the fact that Morgan would be getting glasses at roughly the same age as he had when he was a child.

I surprised him by letting him know that Morgan did not need glasses, but that she needed vision therapy. I tried my best to tell him what the doctor said. I just wanted to sit down and have lunch downtown with my family. Morgan was so happy to be having lunch with her dad close to where he worked.

I just wanted an hour to do something other than think about everything Morgan had to deal with. It was overwhelming for me to think of everything that she had to deal with, imagine what it must be like for her?

I had only worked at the camp for disabled children a few months when I was informed that due to budget cuts my position would no longer be there.

In the short time that I was at the camp, I did learn quite a bit about children with disabilities. I really wanted to understand more about the issues that my daughter was facing, and how I could best help her in this complicated world.

I wondered if by chance this short-lived job could have been a clue into my daughter's issues. I often wondered if she had mild cerebral palsy, I had wondered but later ruled out if she had some form of muscular dystrophy. My nephew had Duchenne's muscular dystrophy, so I knew it was in the family genes somewhere.

I was on the phone with my sister Diane one day and told her that since my extensive work experience at the camp for disabled children (pun intended) and my limited research, the only thing that I could rule out is diabetes.

I did not say this with malice. Diane knew too well what it was like to deal with a diabetic child, she had a young son that had been diabetic since age nine.

I knew that Diane knew what I was talking about. The confusion, the stress, the not knowing but knowing that there was something. Diane, sensing my stress level knowing that I was at my wits end, sent Morgan a letter where she had written each word in a different colour. Yes, that was one of the tricks that I had learnt in vision therapy.

It was now October 2002 and Dr. Wong had managed somehow to get us back into the developmental clinic for the third time. Well, there is the saying, "third time's a charm".

Scott knew how frustrated I was with the previous two experiences at the developmental clinic. So, he came with me.

Again, she saw occupational therapists, physical therapists, child development specialists but the person that really stood out to me was the child psychologist that met with Morgan.

We were not permitted to be in the room with Morgan and the psychologist, but we were able to sit behind a mirror that allowed us to see everything in the room without Morgan being aware of the fact that we could see her.

In my opinion, Morgan answered the questions posed to her in an age-appropriate manner. She was cooperative and quite engaged with this woman.

This third time was different, as we were told that all the therapists and specialists would get together and review everything.

We would come back to meet with them to review their findings, however before we left the child psychologist mentioned how inappropriate she thought Morgan was for sniffling.

Morgan had a bit of a cold at the time, and she sniffled in rather than let her nose drip. The psychologist said that it was highly inappropriate for Morgan to sniffle especially because she had asked her if she had wanted to use a tissue.

I was taken aback by this comment, we were talking about a seven year old child, not an adult. I was so upset by the whole experience; I just wanted to get out of there.

Perhaps I was fixated on this woman's idea of inappropriateness for a seven-year-old child to sniffle in rather than let her nose run or use a tissue, but at this point, my frustration with the whole system was difficult for me to hide.

On my next visit to Dr. Wong, I mentioned what the child psychologist had said about the sniffles and he himself could not believe it.

I told him about all the specialists that Morgan had met that day and he felt confident that we would now be getting the assistance we needed.

I kept thinking how nice it would be to have access to publicly funded occupational therapy, physical therapy, and vision therapy.

I was so excited and hopeful on how a team of specialists assigned to my daughter would help her make progress.

About a month later, we were back at the developmental clinic. I felt comforted that Dr. Wong was there. He went into the boardroom before we did and then we were ushered in.

It was just such a cold and callous environment. We saw the therapists and specialists that Morgan had met with the previous month. There were so many other people sitting in this huge boardroom. It was impossible to keep track of everyone even after they introduced themselves'

I kept wondering, why are there so many people in the room? What's wrong with Morgan? I could feel my heart race and I was so happy that Scott was beside me.

One by one, the specialists described their findings and none of them were positive, none of them were uplifting or encouraging. Of course, the child psychologist lamented about her sniffling, for god's sake woman give that up.

The physical therapist went on and on about what trouble Morgan had with her gait and how she had difficulty catching and throwing a ball.

The occupational therapist was astounded at how delayed Morgan's fine motor skills were. And so, it went on and on. Each person exclaimed about how behind Morgan was.

The end result is that they felt that Morgan had a learning disability that seriously impacted her motor skills.

There were so many times that I wanted to scream at the top of my lungs. I wanted to tell them that they had this negative stuff to say but no clear ideas on how to help Morgan. I wanted to ask why in the previous two visits did no one notice all these issues?

It is hard to hear other people criticize your child, but that was not what was motivating my anger. I desperately tried to get assistance for Morgan, we hired a private occupational therapist, and we worked every single day on her fine motor skills. The last visit at the developmental clinic we were told that her gross motor skills were ahead of her actual age.

Scott could see my anger. He could see me get more frustrated as each person spoke. He kept whispering to me to wait until everything was over.

Sometimes, I am annoyed that I held back. I had a right to be angry at these people who call themselves child specialists, who pretend to care about children in our society. I had been through so much and to sit there and listen to these people was repulsive.

Then Dr. Wong spoke up and he made a reference to the report from the private psychologist that we had seen when Morgan was five years old. He informed them that this psychologist had felt that Morgan had ADHD, and not one of them in that room, after consultation with each other, came up with that diagnosis.

You could see how this information infuriated all of them seated at the table. In essence, they said that they should have been informed of the previous private assessment. Seriously, that's the best they had.

I wondered if they were annoyed at not being told or because they didn't come up with that diagnosis themselves?

I was doing my best to stay calm. Scott certainly was helping me with this, but did it really matter what anyone said? All that really mattered was what was going to be done to help Morgan.

The child development specialist said that they have many wonderful programs for preschoolers, but everything for school aged children was done in the classroom.

I could take no more and left the room. I couldn't believe what just happened. They were saying Morgan would have benefitted from the preschool program that they refused to let her into.

I'm not sure when we were told this, but sometime during the meeting the team said that they would be meeting with the school to ensure that Morgan received the necessary assistance in the classroom and arrange for both occupational therapy and physical therapy in school.

On our way back to Redwood Meadows, I cried. . I was so upset. I felt defeated. I tried so hard to get Morgan the help she needed and now here we were.

I was at home day after day, planning the fine motor skill tasks and working with Morgan on these, inventing games to increase her overall learning and fine motor skills. I was the one doing the work with Morgan many of these times, she did not want to cooperate. She didn't want to sit and do fine motor skill tasks; she was just a kid and wanted to be a kid. I felt so alone at that moment and had really wanted to be close to my family for support.

The following week Scott was out of town on business, but the school/hospital meeting was scheduled, and we couldn't rearrange the date. There were so many people involved and it was extremely difficult to make things work out for everyone's schedule.

I was so happy that Dr. Wong was able to clear his calendar to come to this meeting. Dr. Wong had been a staple in both Morgan and my life since before she turned two and I knew I could count on him.

This meeting was more difficult than I had imagined. Her teacher and the principal and vice-principal and the hospital team, not everyone that was in that giant boardroom from the original meeting, but there was the child development specialist, occupational therapist and physical therapist.

It was just back and forth from both sides, all the negativity one could imagine in that small windowless school meeting room. If it wasn't the school complaining about Morgan's inability to stay within the lines when colouring, it was the hospital saying how behind she was in her ball throwing and so on and so on. Both sides commented on her gait, how it didn't seem right.

I had expected Dr. Wong to step in and say something, but he didn't, he didn't say one word. I was dumbfounded, why had he bothered to come to this meeting, why had he wasted his time here when he was just going to sit there without saying a word. Scott couldn't make the meeting due to him being out of town for work, I had counted on Dr. Wong to support me.

Finally, a lull came in the conversation or bickering or whatever it was and Dr. Wong asked, "Are we finished?" He asked this in a calm fashion. Here he sat quiet throughout the whole thing and now he is asking if they were finished.

There was an acknowledgement by both the school side and the hospital side to indicate that indeed they were finished. He did not miss a beat, in fact he amazed me. I am feeling very guilty about questioning why he had even attended this meeting.

He said, "I have listened to both the school and the hospital talk about the issues at hand, many times they were the same issue being rehashed. Not once have I heard either the school or the hospital talk about what they plan to do to work with Morgan to ensure that she is successful in school and in life!"

You could have heard a pin drop; these ladies' jaws dropped and all of them were put in their place with the words of Dr. Wong. He continued to say that he has known Morgan for five years and he knows what a bright young girl she is and that she has the capacity to be a contributing member of society with some guidance.

He repeated his question now directed at the principal of the school and she said that she would implement the request by the hospital to have both occupational therapy and physical therapy in the school for Morgan. She continued to say that she would discuss with Morgan's teacher and put an IPP (Individual Program Plan) in place and would code Morgan as having a learning disability.

Dr. Wong then asked if this meant that Morgan would be provided with an aid to help her throughout her elementary school years. The principal said that Morgan would have to be coded with a physical disability to have extra help in the classroom.

Dr. Wong asked why the principal could not code Morgan as having a physical disability. He told the principal that he listened to everything that was said by both the school team and the hospital team, and he heard many instances where there were comments about her gait, about her inability to run like the other children and participate in gym. He said that as Morgan's pediatrician he would be happy to supply them with whatever they needed to ensure that there was more help in the classroom for

Morgan. He said that after respectively listening to everyone that he felt that Morgan did have a physical disability and required extra assistance in the classroom.

The principal shot Dr. Wong down and I could see that he had had enough. The meeting came to an end and Dr. Wong had to rush to get back to Calgary, as we walked out of the meeting room, he said to me "run, as fast as you can from this school, they will not help your daughter!"

I hardly had time to digest the conversation from this pessimistic meeting but had to gather my thoughts with the discussion of a physical disability. I had never thought of that. Many people had mentioned Morgan's gait, and certainly, her running was questionable, she certainly was clumsy and awkward, but did she really have a physical disability?

When I next spoke with Dr. Wong, I thanked him for taking the time to go to both the meetings, the first one at the Child Development Clinic and the second one at the school.

Dr. Wong always made me feel good. He told me that had I not worked with Morgan as diligently as I had that she would not be able to do half the things that she was doing.

He told me that it was extremely easy for the school to code Morgan as having a physical disability with all the information from the hospital and then having him as back up.

He told me that he had no idea why the school did not want to code Morgan in this fashion, but he repeated that this school would never be the right place for Morgan.

I started applying to private schools immediately. Both Scott and I were against sending our daughter to private school. We both wanted her to enjoy going to school with the same children that were in the neighbourhood so that she would see her friends in school and around the community, just as we both had. I continued to worry about Morgan but soon I'd have to worry about myself too.

ELEVEN

MY TURN

Sometime a few weeks after this meeting, I developed severe pain and was vomiting. The pain was too much to bear and although I did not want to go to the hospital, I knew that I had to.

Shortly after Morgan was born, my doctor diagnosed me with severe PMS, some months it wasn't so bad and other months it was hardly bearable. How could I seriously go to the emergency room because I had PMS?

I struggled with the idea for a few hours, as it was nearing Morgan's bedtime, I asked Scott to take me to hospital. I knew I had to go. I didn't want to have to wake her up in the middle of the night, there was no way that I could drive myself there.

Scott couldn't stay at the hospital with me, as we had no one that could help with Morgan, and he had to get her to bed so that she could attend school the next day.

I was in the emergency room and slept on and off that night. Scott took Morgan to school and came to visit with me. The hospital wasn't sure what was wrong but knew that my liver enzymes were out of whack.

I wanted to go home. I wanted to be there when Morgan got home from school. The hospital said that I could go home, but it would be a much longer process for them to discover what was wrong with me.

The doctor told me that it was not simply PMS and that it was something way more serious than that. Scott told me that it would be best for me to stay in the hospital so, I stayed. Of course, I was nervous, but I was more concerned about Morgan and how she would be able to understand why her mom wasn't at home waiting for her.

Scott stayed at the hospital until he had to go to pick up Morgan. At times like this when things are so uncertain it would be nice to have family around. I had no family around. I had no one I could count on. No one could go and pick Morgan up from school and let her spend the weekend with. No one came and visited while Scott went to pick up Morgan from school, there was no one.

Scott drove to Bragg Creek to pick Morgan up from school and brought her to the hospital to visit. I was so worried that Morgan would be overly concerned about me being in the hospital. What does a seven-year-old know about these types of things? I had never been sick or in the hospital before. I could only imagine what was going through her mind.

I needed her to see me so that she could see that I was ok. By this time I was feeling much better. Of course, the morphine drip could have been part of it.

I enjoyed seeing Morgan, it was as if I hadn't seen her in months and literally it hadn't been a full 24 hours. She was curious about the hospital beds but loved all the attention that this pretty little seven-year-old garnered by all the nurses on the unit.

Shortly after Morgan arrived, a doctor walked in. He asked the nurse if she could take Morgan to the nurse's station and show her around.

I knew at this point that the doctor had something serious to discuss with me. What could it be? I had never been sick, yet his demeanor told me I should be concerned.

Scott and I sat at the edge of the hospital bed and the doctor was leaning in towards us and he asked, "Now be honest with me, how much alcohol do you consume in a day?"

Scott and I looked at each other in dismay, alcohol, I am a teetotaler.

"I don't drink any alcohol ever," I responded right away. The doctor looked perplexed; I could tell that he was hoping that I would say that I was a heavy drinker. I think this would have solved the problem. I think this would have been so much easier on him in terms of a diagnosis.

At this point, he came closer to us. Now all three of us were sitting on the hospital bed. He replies that if I am not a drinker then he believes that I have liver cancer, but he wanted to rule out something first.

He had had one patient before that had a gallbladder issue that persisted so long that it turned to mush and that this mush had negatively impacted the liver, he did caution us and said that he had only seen this one time and he is leaning towards liver cancer.

What can you say when you are told that you probably have cancer? It was unreal. How could this even be possible? My mind was racing.

I was grasping at straws, and I knew it, but I did tell him that shortly after

the birth of my daughter, I had had issues that my doctor explained as PMS.

I told him that the symptoms always seemed to occur roughly a week prior to my menstrual cycle. I did explain that the pain and discomfort and sometimes vomiting occurred regardless of what I ate.

He was a compassionate man and told us not to worry too much, that he was putting in a rush request to go to another hospital to run a special test.

The doctor left the room and in ran Morgan. Scott and I did not have time to discuss or even digest what the doctor had just said.

There was no way that either of us were going to discuss cancer in front of Morgan. Shortly after the doctor left Scott and Morgan headed home. While the talk with the doctor left me incredibly perplexed, I knew that Scott had a more difficult journey as he not only had to digest this information, but he also had to take care of a very precocious seven year old girl.

I was now all alone in the hospital bed. I don't ever remember feeling so alone. My family were all in eastern Canada. I was alone to contemplate the words the doctor had said, those words would not leave me alone. They were there even when I tried to ignore them. "I believe that you have liver cancer!" I wanted those words to disappear. I want this whole thing to be gone.

I tried unsuccessfully to get lost in a T.V. show. I wanted something, anything to take my mind off those horrible words.

I wanted to be able to talk to someone that I love. I didn't want to face this diagnosis on my own. Scott needed to be with Morgan. I understood that, but I was alone.

Of course, Scott told his family, but no one offered to take Morgan so that he could be with me at the hospital.

Nighttime was upon me; I can't even count how many times the words liver cancer danced in my head. I have never been overly religious, I mean as a child in rural Quebec, we were forced to attend Sunday school and church on a weekly basis, but I had long left that behind me.

That night sitting alone in my hospital bed I said a prayer......." Lord, please help me and my family. I understand that things in the world happen as they are supposed to happen and that you have a reason for everything. If you feel that I must endure cancer, please don't let it be now when my daughter is only seven years old, she needs me!"

Praying at that time made me think of a scene from the movie Bruce Almighty with Morgan Freeman and Jim Carrey. The scene where Jim Carrey's character must respond to prayers from his computer, he gets his coffee filled by Juan Valdez and starts typing away, originally having 1,527,503 prayers to answer.

After feverishly typing away, he refreshes the page and now has over 3,500,000 prayers to answer. He simply presses "yes" to every prayer. I guess you had to see the movie, but seriously, with so much going on in the world, did I really expect God to take away liver cancer?

Early the next morning the nurse ran into my room and said that I was not going to have breakfast as they arranged for me to take a test at another hospital. This was Saturday, and I couldn't believe that they were able to get me in. This only deepened my thought that I did indeed have liver cancer. Why else would they rush this procedure?

I phoned Scott to let him know and he feverishly tried to find someone to take care of Morgan. He finally reached his dad and was able to bring Morgan to where his Dad had been staying with a friend in Cochrane, then he hurried over to the hospital.

When I woke up at the hospital, Scott was there. I was still groggy from the anesthetic, but it was nice to have Scott there. My first question was "Where is Morgan"? She was always at the forefront of my thoughts, always.

Later that afternoon, the doctor came to my room and said that I needed emergency surgery to remove my gallbladder. Yes, remove my gallbladder, I did not have liver cancer.

Of course, he went on to explain what was happening and why they could not detect issues with my gallbladder and how it is a rare occurrence. Honestly, I don't remember much of what was said. I just wanted to have my gallbladder removed and carry on.

On Sunday Morning I had the surgery and Scott and Morgan visited me later that evening. It was so nice to see Morgan, how difficult it must be for her, not to understand what was happening to her mother. That wasn't as important as the fact that I did not have liver cancer.

I remained in the hospital overnight and Monday morning Scott and Morgan came to pick me up to bring me home. Scott kept Morgan from school so that she could be part of the homecoming. I'm sure that school would not have been a good place for her that day anyhow.

Now onto the road of recovery, I shifted my thoughts back to Morgan and our idea of a private school.

I needed to be strong to prepare for the fight ahead. There always seemed to be a fight ahead. It wasn't that I wanted one, I didn't. I wanted Morgan to get what she needed, and it never came without a struggle.

TWELVE

ONLY THREE RIDES

I was on top of everything at school. I was now at home full time, believe me I was busier than most moms who worked full time. I was asking the school about occupational therapy and physical therapy; I questioned everything written in Morgan's IPP plan at school. I invented and created different games to help Morgan with her schoolwork as well as the delays in her motor skills.

Here comes the real shocker. The school occupational therapist said that at most she could visit with Morgan was once a month for half an hour. The teacher felt that all the students would benefit from having an occupational therapist in the classroom so instead of having just Morgan work with the occupational therapist, she joined the classroom.

The school physical therapist felt that Morgan's gross motor skills were only slightly behind, despite the report from the developmental clinic. As a result, due to the case load he was unable to travel to Bragg Creek to work with Morgan. Totally unbelievable and totally unacceptable, but that is what I had to work with.

Scott and I agreed that we had to do everything possible to help Morgan in spite of the cost. We had already been working with a private occupational therapist and were now working with a private vision therapist. We saw the vision therapist once a week and we alternated weeks between spending time with the private physical therapist and the private occupational therapist.

Every Thursday afternoon, I would pick Morgan up early from school and we would head for work with the vision therapist and depending on the week would continue with either the physical therapist or the occupational therapist. Keep in mind that none of these therapies were covered by the public health system, not one of them.

At home, we worked steadfastly every day with Morgan on her three therapies. We were determined to help her succeed, but it wasn't always easy.

What kid wants to work continuously on these therapies? I had to do extra work to ensure that she had some fun while working on her motor skills. Other than the games that I created to help her learn to spell and with her math, I would take every opportunity to make sure that she was working on her motor skills without even knowing that she was. Seriously, as a child ages, motor skill therapy becomes a tedious chore.

For Halloween that year, I bought brown paper lunch bags as Halloween treat bags. Every day after school we would decorate each bag to give to the trick or treaters on Halloween night.

I would have Morgan trace witches and ghosts onto the bags and then she would have to colour them. She so enjoyed this and had no idea that it was really something we were doing to improve her fine motor skills.

You could say that by now I had developed a schedule that Morgan followed every day after school. She would have a snack, then we would go outside and play. She needed to have some physical activity before we could concentrate on anything else.

Depending on the day, we would either bounce on the trampoline, to help her with her balance, or we would throw a big ball to each other, or play a game of one-on-one soccer.

After she was worn out, we would work on her vision exercises, and then onto homework and fine motor skill work, often combining the two with the games that I had created for her.

By the time Scott came home for supper we had completed most of her exercises, however, we always took the opportunity to help her with all her motor skills delays with whatever we were doing.

Scott loved hockey and enjoyed playing weekly with friends and clients in the oil and gas industry. For two years straight while we were living in Redwood Meadows, he built a small rink on the side of our home.

Morgan loved this time spent with her dad. We quickly realized that Morgan was not going to be a skater. Scott tried to encourage her to put on her skates while they went outdoors on the rink to play hockey.

She loved being on the rink and she loved to play hockey, she just didn't want anything to do with skates. She loved the crisp fresh air on her cheeks, but no thank you, skating was not for her.

We were coming to the end of grade two when I got the call from the private school. We set up an appointment time for us to meet the following week.

How would I bring this subject up to Morgan, by now, she was singing the school song and felt a belonging to a place that did not feel the same way about her?

The innocence of a child is beautiful, but I was her mom. I saw that the public school did nothing to help her.

A few weeks before the private school called, after a particularly difficult day at school, Morgan, now eight years old, said to me "Mom, I want to cut off my hands so new hands that work better can grow!"

Holy shit, I knew that school was tough for Morgan. I knew that she had difficulty keeping up with the other kids mainly due to the difficulty that she experienced with fine motor skills, but to hear her talk like that was a punch in the gut.

I'm her mother. I felt like a failure. I've tried everything to make it better for her. I'm there to protect her and she now wants to cut her hands off.

I spoke with Morgan and explained that if she cut off her hands that new hands would not grow back, just that she would have no hands and quite possibly die because of the loss of blood.

I told her that I was looking at another school that had less children in each classroom and more teachers. I didn't want to say too much. I had no idea if she was going to be accepted into the private school.

We were continuously disappointed by the very institutions that were set up to help. So, I wanted to make sure that Morgan didn't feel sad or disappointed if she wasn't accepted to the private school.

The appointment was upon us. We met with a counselor, and she said that she would do some testing with Morgan to determine if they felt that they could help her.

I was nervous, my stomach was in knots. I kept thinking and thinking about how far Morgan had come.

I knew that she was bright and anyone that had a conversation with her always assumed she was older than her age. I was open and honest with the school about Morgan's motor skill delays.

I wanted to be sure that they were in a good position to help her with this. Certainly, I had only heard wonderful things about the school and felt confident that they were aptly suited to work with children like Morgan. Bright children that just needed more one on one attention.

I watched as the counselor and Morgan walked towards me down a long corridor. They were chatting up a storm and both seemed to be enjoying themselves.

Morgan, who was just finishing up grade two, had impressed the counselor with reading grade eleven words. I was so happy. We worked so hard with the vision therapy and the daily exercises, and it seemed to have paid off.

Morgan, who at the end of grade one, could not read at a grade one level was now at the end of grade two reading at a grade eleven level! Talk about a proud mama. Of course, Morgan was accepted into the private school.

Both Scott and I were so excited to know that Morgan would be out of that public school that didn't want to help her. I say "didn't" want to help her because they could have, they could have coded her as having a physical disability as the hospital and Dr. Wong had indicated but they refused to do so. Morgan could have had a full-time attendant at school to help her with her daily tasks potentially alleviating some of the stress she experienced every day.

We were hopeful and knew that we had to move forward, not backwards, it wouldn't serve any good for Morgan for us to focus on the past.

We were so excited that the vision therapy, while expensive, was helping. We were disappointed that neither the occupational therapy nor physical therapy were having the same positive results.

But we persevered, every day during the summer, I worked with Morgan on vision therapy, physical therapy, and occupational therapy. It was evident that Morgan lagged more in her fine motor skills than her gross motor skills, so we really worked on these.

Summer between grade two and three was upon us but we did not relax. We worked every day on all areas to help Morgan prepare for grade three.

We lived close to Calaway Park. We had been there a few times when Morgan was younger. This year we bought a season pass. I wanted to make sure she had fun during her summer vacation and not only the therapies.

We got to the park just before it opened and there were so many kids waiting at the entrance. It was already warm, but I was excited to spend the day with Morgan and to watch her enjoy the rides.

Finally, the gates opened and with our season pass, Morgan could go on every ride in kiddy land as many times as she liked.

I noticed a lot of kids rushing to different rides and I asked Morgan which ride she wanted to go on first. She looked at me and then looked over at some rides and said "Mom, I have to look at the rides first. I can only go on three rides, so I want to pick my favourite three."

I immediately assumed that Morgan misunderstood, we were going to spend the entire day at the amusement park she wasn't limited to three rides.

Morgan told me that she couldn't stay at Calaway Park for more than three rides, as it hurts her too much to do all that walking.

To say that I was shocked was an understatement. I remembered she had complained of hip pain, and she even told me that was the reason she had to sit in the shopping cart when we went to Chinook Mall, but here we were at Calaway Park, a local well respected amusement park, how could she have concerns here.

At that moment, I knew this was way more serious than I ever thought. What eight-year-old kid is going to say that they can only do three rides, when they're told that they can go on all the rides?

This did not make sense and I knew that a call to Dr. Wong was in order.

Dr. Wong checked Morgan's hips and legs and could not detect anything. He reviewed all the reports that he received from the developmental clinic. They had met with Morgan on three occasions and on the last occasion, it appeared as if they had done a thorough check up of her.

He looked at me and said that perhaps Morgan should be assessed by a Neurologist. Great, I thought, just another thing to add to the list, another stressor in our already strained lives.

What was wrong with Morgan? I was so very worried about her and Dr. Wong was extremely sympathetic but couldn't find any reason why she could only do the three rides.

Although I always tried to be positive, as a mother I knew something was very wrong.

Grade three was upon us and Morgan was a little concerned about it. It was a new school to her. It was going to be different not to be with the children that she knew from the school near Redwood Meadows.

I explained to her that although she had the same teacher for grades one and two, that she would have had a different teacher in grade three even if she remained at the local school.

My past experiences with the school system had left a bad impression on me. I naively expected them to do more. My faith was somewhat renewed when I met Morgan's new teacher at the private school.

There was a total of 15 children in the classroom and the teacher had two assistants that worked with her. Morgan felt right at home because of this incredible woman.

Morgan soared; her confidence level was at an all time high. I had never seen her beam so much after school. I was so happy and felt that we finally found the right place for Morgan, and she would succeed.

A few months after school started, we were in to meet with the Neurologist. I was so hesitant to even keep the appointment, not because I didn't think Morgan needed to see someone. I knew that something wasn't right, and it was having an impact on Morgan's mobility, but a neurologist?

THIRTEEN

ARE WE MISSING SOMETHING?

The child neurologist greeted us warmly. He seemed to be such a warm and welcoming individual, all my apprehension went out the window. This man seemed to generally care for children, could this be another Dr. Wong?

He told me that he had reviewed the now infamous reports from the developmental clinic, so I knew that he understood the situation. I explained that the reason for our visit was that Morgan had been complaining of hip pain as far back as age five, but that more recently it seemed to be more serious.

I explained about needing to use a shopping cart for Morgan to sit in while going through a mall. I mentioned the situation at the amusement park and told him that many therapists had commented about her gait.

I gave him a brief run down of the delays that Morgan had encountered in her life. I told him how much work we had been doing with private therapists to help Morgan with her motor skills. I beamed when I told him about how she was so positive about the private school she was attending and that I couldn't have imagined how much this school had changed her overall demeanour.

The neurologist had Morgan do some tasks, such as ride a giant tricycle, which was much beneath her now that she was using a two-wheel bike. He had her run back and forth, he had her walk on her tiptoes, he had her throw and catch a ball. But then, he just spoke with her, like he was her best friend, asked about school, about her hobbies etc. They both seemed to be enjoying the conversation.

I nervously waited to hear what this Doctor would say. Obviously, something was wrong, but what? I had only started to feel a little better about Morgan's progress because of the private school. I dreaded that I would hear anything that would dampen this spirit.

The neurologist turned to me and said "Mom, you've done a phenomenal job with this young girl!" Oh my God, did he just say that? I didn't realize that I needed someone to tell me that. I needed to feel that all the work was fruitful. I had validation for all the work that I had done, and I needed that validation, but at what cost?

He went on to say that based on what he had read, he was super impressed with how well Morgan was doing and that he had no concerns whatsoever.

I was on cloud 9. Morgan was doing well in school and loving it. The neurologist said that everything was fine. Could we finally relax? Is the worst of it over? I knew I shouldn't question what the neurologist said, I should be so happy that nothing is wrong. Why am I feeling uncomfortable with the statement from the neurologist, why can't I just accept that nothing is wrong and go forward with it. Nothing was wrong, everything was ok. I desperately tried to shove Morgan's hip and mobility issues to the back of my mind, because nothing was wrong. How many more times did I need to hear this to believe it.

Scott was very happy to hear that everything was fine, he said that he was happy that now we could relax and live a more normal life.

By the time grade four started, we had stopped all the therapies for a few reasons, vision therapy was a success, and we weren't required to continue with it. Occupational therapy and physical therapy were not giving us as great a result as the vision therapy had. With all the work we had been doing at home and now the school seemed to be helping in these areas, we decided to stop them all. Afterall, we were now forced to pay private school fees for Morgan, on just one income. I continued all my work with

Morgan to help her with both her fine motor skills and her gross motor skills.

Grade four turned into grade five. Morgan seemed to be more like every other kid. What a relief for her not to have to go to vision therapy, occupational therapy, or physical therapy. She was growing leaps and bounds and was developing such incredible friendships.

I wasn't fooling myself; I knew that something wasn't "right" for a lack of a better word. I was certainly over the moon happy with what the neurologist had told me, yet, as a mother, I felt that we were all missing something. There was something, just what it was I wasn't sure. Morgan still had difficulty with walking a great distance and her gait was different from most kids her age, but I tried my best to put everything behind us. Morgan was fine, the neurologist told me so.

FOURTEEN

DEALING WITH THE WAIT

Dr. Wong had always told me that he believed that "mothers know", and here we were with a diagnosis of severe scoliosis. I was reeling over the idiotic words that the nurse had just told me.
"**SCOLIOSIS DOES NOT HURT!**"
Even after explaining to her that the only way we discovered that Morgan had scoliosis was due to the pain. How could she utter such an insensitive statement?

I thought long and hard and wondered what I should do. I couldn't give up, Morgan still needed me to fight for her. Did I have any fight left? Of course, I did. I am her mother and there was no way that I was going to let an orthopaedic nurse discourage me from fighting for my daughter. I needed to keep fighting, there had to be a way to get Morgan the help she needed.

After this call, I decided to reach out to my MLA. This was a different MLA, as I was now living in the west end of Calgary. I knew the drill; I had done this before. I was prepared to keep calling and keep bothering the people in his office, because I was not giving up.

I left my first message at my MLA's office and to my surprise a few days later he called back. It totally caught me off guard, this did not happen the last time and I was dumbfounded when he called. As briefly as I could, I explained the long and frustrating health care journey that we had been on. I spoke of the neurologist appointment when she was 8 years old and how now that she is 11 years old, she had severe scoliosis and we are told that she will have to wait an undetermined amount of time for surgery.

The MLA said that he was going to contact the head of the health region and that someone would get back to me shortly. I understood that he felt he had to say something. I felt that no one was going to get back to me. I've played this game a bit too long. I was all too familiar with how things really worked.

Two weeks later, I got a call from a woman indicating that she was with the health region and that my MLA had asked her to reach out to me. Now I am in disbelief. Someone pinch me. I could not believe that someone from the health region had reached out to me, it's unbelievable.

We set up an appointment to meet. To my surprise, we met next door to the orthopaedic unit. At this point, I did not care who's feathers I ruffled, or what anyone thought of me. I am her voice and I had to fight for her.

I was so very prepared for the meeting. I wasn't going to hold anything back. I was fed up with just accepting what I was told by various health care professionals.

This woman actually listened to me. I told her of the appointments and lack of action from the developmental clinic. I told her of the fact that we couldn't get occupational therapy or physical therapy in the school.

I explained about the issues with the hip pain and Morgan's inability to walk too far. I told her that the neurologist had given me false reassurance that nothing was wrong with Morgan. I let her know how rude and demeaning the nurse in the orthopedic unit was and how without Dr. Wong in the picture I was struggling to find my way through this maze.

Now here we were at age 11, Morgan had a 52-degree left side curve and I was extremely worried about her heart and lungs. I stressed upon her that the wait or the uncertainty was very difficult for Morgan and although she doesn't verbalize it, I knew that she was very anxious about the surgery. The not knowing was extremely difficult for her. Who was I kidding? The uncertainty of everything was making me sick. I knew it, but I also knew that I had to fight for her! I was so hopeful that she would hear our story and understand everything that we had gone through and put

Morgan at the top of the list for surgery. Of course, that was a pipe dream to say the least. All she said was that the issues were noted, and that Morgan would be placed in the order in which her surgery was deemed necessary.

I was lost for words! After everything I just told this woman she had the audacity to tell me that "Morgan would be placed in the order in which her surgery was deemed necessary." Did she not hear a word I said?

To my surprise a few weeks later the MLA called me to find out how my meeting went with the representative from the health region. When I got over the shock of the fact that he was actually calling me back. I responded that I felt as if my meeting with the health region representative was a total waste of time.

He seemed surprised by my comments and said that he would see to it that something was done to ensure that Morgan got proper health care. Yeah, right, I had heard that line so many times and I had never seen any results from it.

At our next appointment, mid October 2006, with the orthopaedic surgeon, I noticed a slight change in his demeanor. He indicated that he understood my concerns about Morgan's scoliosis and that while he still believed her scoliosis to be idiopathic in nature, he referred her to visit with yet another neurologist.

I still held a lot of resentment towards the neurologist that had assured me that nothing was wrong with Morgan when she was 8 years old. Yet he had noted and failed to tell me that she had scoliosis back then. I was a bit jaded with the idea of visiting another neurologist based on this encounter.

In addition to announcing that Morgan would be visiting with a different neurologist, he mentioned that her spinal fusion surgery would be in May 2007.

Still far away, but he noted that her scoliosis curve was increasing 2 degrees a month and there was some concern about her heart.

Just what every mother wants to hear, that the scoliosis is increasing faster than doctors would expect and that since it is on her left side they were concerned about her heart. I am even more overwhelmed than before. I don't want to hear this; I don't want to believe this. This is all too much for me.

The final interesting moment was when the orthopaedic surgeon introduced Morgan and me to a different nurse. Aha, perhaps, my talk with the health region representative did have some impact. I was extremely thankful that I would not have to deal with the nurse that was so rude and condescending.

May 2007 seemed so far away. How could a child live day by day, going to school, hanging with friends knowing that she would be having this major surgery? I was still amazed that any child would have to wait so long for surgery, especially with the doctor's comments about the curve's progression and the possible impact on her heart.

We met with the neurologist that the orthopaedic surgeon referred us to, she asked a million questions about Morgan's early development, ordered several x-rays and blood tests, but she too said that everything was fine.

At this point, those were only words with no real meaning.

FIFTEEN

SPINAL FUSION

By the time March 2007 rolled around, Morgan, Scott and I were anxious, nervous, and stressed about the upcoming surgery. It felt as if there were a heaviness on us that we could not explain. Perhaps parents in similar shoes would understand, but no one else could ever understand this heaviness.

It was around this time that I mentioned to nurse number two that Morgan was having difficulty sleeping. The nurse looked at us in amazement, and responded to my concerns "Oh, did no one mention that we have a psychologist in the orthopedic department that Morgan can access to discuss her concerns about scoliosis and the upcoming surgery?"

Unbelievable, seriously unbelievable! Imagine a psychologist who deals with children that are experiencing orthopedic issues and surgeries and this is the first time we've been made aware of this? Her surgery was less than 3 months away and now they tell us?

Thankfully, Morgan met with the psychologist the following week and by all accounts it went well. Morgan had weekly appointments with the psychologist, and she looked forward to these appointments. Although the appointments did not help with Morgan's sleeping issues, it was evident that Morgan felt more comfortable about herself and the upcoming surgery after each visit.

During our April 2007 appointment with the orthopaedic surgeon, he announced that Morgan's surgery date was May 30th. We were given a tour of the hospital and what to expect while Morgan was an in-patient. Here we were about a month away from the big date and it seemed too close. How ironic, we tried to have the surgery as soon as possible so that Morgan could move on, yet here we were, and it seemed too close. Certainly, this was just my fear talking. I knew that we had to get this done and over with, but were we ready? Can any parent ever be ready knowing that their child has to go through a spinal fusion surgery?

During this appointment, Morgan asked the surgeon how long the surgery would be. The response he gave put a smile on Scott's and my face, but I believe it went over Morgan's head.

He responded, "Well Morgan, it depends on who you are. For you, it will seem like a minute of two, because you will be asleep during the procedure. For your parents, it will seem like a lifetime, but for me it will be about 8 hours."

Although we knew that Morgan would make a full recovery from her surgery, Scott and I thought that with the ever so minor risk of paralysis, it would be a good idea to take Morgan to Disneyland. To let her enjoy the rides and the whole experience. Besides, we thought that it would be a great distraction for her with the surgery just weeks away.

We pulled Morgan from school, hopped on a plane that first landed in Denver and then headed to Los Angeles. We were living in the 4th largest city in Canada with a population of just over 1.2 million people, the population of Los Angeles was about 4 times the population of Calgary, needless to say, I left all the driving up to Scott.

Morgan and Scott were delighted as the third film of the Pirates of the Caribbean, At World's End, was being released that month and there was much fanfare at Disneyland supporting this movie. This movie was the highest grossing film of 2007 and earned Academy Award nominations for best makeup and for best visual effects. Many Pirates of the Caribbean souvenirs were taken home with us.

There were the obvious rides with Splash Mountain being one of the all-time favourites. Of course, we got to see Mickey and Minnie and so many of the Disney Princesses.

Morgan enjoyed Disneyland immensely although she did have some difficulty with the walking and standing in lines because of the back and hip pain. Nonetheless, this excursion to Disneyland certainly helped to ease our tensions regarding the upcoming surgery.

Impossible to totally forget that shortly Morgan would be having a spinal fusion. Seriously, a spinal fusion is surgery that permanently connects two or more vertebrae in the spine, eliminating motion between them. Metal plates, screws and rods are usually used to hold the vertebrae together.

Definitely sounds wonderful, I don't want to think about this for too long. I mustn't dwell on things I can't change. Morgan must have this surgery, the surgeon said so. I am very worried about the impact on her heart and lungs.

The morning of May 30th was upon us, needless to say no one in the house got very much sleep the night before. But it was here, the day that we had thought we wanted, but did we really? Did we really understand the dynamics of what a spinal fusion was and how this could impact our daughter's life?

We were feeling so lost, but we had to rely on the advice of the orthopaedic surgeon. We were very concerned about the curve hitting her heart. Our daughter's life was literally in someone else's hands.

We arrived at the surgical ward and were greeted by a few nurses. They asked Morgan to change into a gown and to wait on a stretcher for the anaesthesiologist. Morgan was truly amazing, she put on a brave face, but we knew that she was extremely nervous.

She was pacing up and down the hallway and asking questions of the nurses. Often, she repeated some of the questions. I wasn't sure if this was because she was nervous or wanted to see if the nurses would give her the same answer.

Time was ticking away, it seemed like hours, but obviously it was mere minutes. The surgeon walked into the area and Morgan was dancing up a storm. She was literally dancing, I'm sure it was just to help her deal with the stress, but the surgeon was quite impressed with her dancing and screamed "Way to go Morgan, that's what I like to see, give me a high five!" You could see some of the fear in Morgan's face subside as she gave the surgeon a high five.

The surgeon proceeded to tell Morgan about the anaesthetic and what would be happening to her before he started to straighten her spine. I am not sure what Morgan heard or understood, all I know is that I really didn't want to hear any of it.

I just wanted Morgan to go into surgery and come back like new. No more back pain, no more rib hump, no more concern about her heart and lungs. As the surgeon so eloquently put it, "after surgery, it will be as if you never had scoliosis!"

The anaesthesiologist arrived and began explaining to Morgan what his role was during the surgery. I kept wondering why on earth are they explaining everything to her, it seemed to just raise her anxiety about the whole thing. Just do it and get it over with. At this point, all we want is for the surgery to be over with.

The anaesthesiologist allowed Scott and me to be with Morgan right up until she was under general anaesthetic. While I was hoping that this helped Morgan feel better knowing that her parents were with her right up until she was under, it was a horrible experience for Scott and me.

One moment she was up and dancing around like a normal pre-teen girl and the next moment she looked like a corpse.

Now the waiting began. Scott and I were on edge, it was the most difficult thing either one of us had gone through. We needed to be with each other for support, yet we needed to be away from each other as we handled stress differently.

As I sat and sat for what seemed like an eternity in the waiting room, I started to write in a journal. I wrote as if I were speaking with Morgan, and she could hear me. The first entry read "Morgan it is almost 10 a.m., we haven't heard anything, and they say no news is good news, so I am hoping that all is going well with you. I want you to know that I am thinking of you, and I love you so much."

It did seem a bit odd to be writing to your child in a journal while she was undergoing surgery, but it helped me. I needed anything that could help me cope. I also brought along a book and a scarf to knit. I am not much of a knitter, I always envied how my mom could knit such beautiful sweaters, hats, mittens and scarfs.

I was not nearly as good a knitter as she was, but I needed things to keep my mind busy. My daughter was having a spinal fusion and it would last at least 8 hours. I needed to keep busy.

Before I discovered that my daughter had scoliosis, I had no clue what a spinal fusion was; the website Spine-Health.com explains it as follows.

"There are several variations to spinal fusion surgery for scoliosis, but most use modern instrumentation systems in which hooks, and screws are applied to the spine to anchor long rods. The surgeon then:

- Uses the rods to carefully reposition the spine at the segments affected by scoliosis, correcting the abnormal rotation and reducing the lateral (sideways) curvature; and
- Grafts bone to the vertebral segments that are to be fused. These bone grafts typically come from a donor or bone bank or part of the patient's own bone such as from the patient's hip. In recent years, there have also been some bone grafts using synthetic bone substitutes; however, long term results and potential risks are not yet fully known.

The rods are essentially used as a splint to hold the spine in place while the bones continue to fuse after surgery is completed. The initial fusion process usually takes about 3 to 6 months, and the fusion will usually continue to take hold for up to 12 months.

Once the fusion has set up, the spine's shape and position are held in place by its long, newly fused bone (not the rods). The rods are generally not removed since this would be a large and unnecessary surgery. Occasionally, a rod can irritate the soft tissue around the spine, in which case the rod can be removed without affecting the fused spine's stability."[4]

---

[4] <u>https://www.spine-health.com/treatment/back-surgery/spinal-fusion-idiopathic-scoliosis</u>

The stress of just sitting in that room surrounded by other parents and family members equally stressed as they waited for their loved ones was more than I could handle.

I kept seeing nurses and doctors coming into the waiting room and either telling the parents that everything was going well but that they are still in surgery or that the surgery was completed. No one was coming to tell Scott and me that Morgan's surgery was going well and/or that it was completed.

Nonsense I thought to myself. I know that Morgan's surgery is not over. We were told it would be at least 8 hours, but how I wished someone would come to let me know that everything was going well.

As the afternoon came and went, I saw so many parents leave the waiting room. I lost myself. I felt as if I were in the waiting room physically but that I really wasn't there spiritually.

I felt as if I were floating above the parents that remained in the waiting area and seeing their stress and feeling as if all their stress was entering my body, as if I didn't have enough stress of my own.

The stress was so overwhelming that Scott and I could barely speak to each other. We fed off each other's stress which actually seemed to make it worse. Scott would go for a brief walk every hour or so. He encouraged me to leave the waiting area and go outside or even to the cafeteria, but I didn't want to leave that waiting room.

I kept thinking that maybe, just maybe someone would come to let me know that Morgan was doing ok. I certainly did not want to be out taking a walk when they came. No matter how long I waited, no one came.

Around 7 p.m. on the intercom system we heard "would the parents of Morgan please meet up with her in the intensive care unit!"

My heart was pounding. We were told that someone would let us know when the surgery was over, and they didn't. Now she is in the ICU!

Scoliosis Does Not Hurt

How long ago did the surgery end? How long was she in the recovery area? Why didn't someone come and tell us that the surgery was over? Leaving us to wait until 7 p.m. was unfathomable.

I tried to get up to get to the elevator, but my legs didn't work. They felt like jelly, and I needed Scott's assistance to get out of the chair. It was evident what the stress of the day had on my body.

We rushed to get to the ICU unit to see Morgan. To see your child hooked up to so many machines was more unbearable than most parents could manage.

Scott and I glanced at all the tubes and heard all the beeps and then glanced at each other, neither one of us were prepared for this.

We definitely did not want Morgan to see our concern, we wanted to have a happy smiley type face so that she wouldn't be as upset by the situation as we were.

The first thing that Morgan said was "Mom, Dad, I don't have that back pain anymore!" That was terrific, that was our end goal. I wished the nurses in the ICU would report this statement back to the orthopaedic unit. I so wish that the efficient nurse number one in the orthopaedic unit would have been in earshot of Morgan that day to hear that yes scoliosis can and does hurt.

As medical professionals, they were fully aware that it could cause pain. The insensitivity of that nurse still bothered me a lot. I wanted her to hear Morgan at this moment so she wouldn't make another child or parent feel terrible when they explained how badly scoliosis hurt.

Morgan woke just long enough to let us know that she did not have anymore "of that" back pain. I'm sure that she had significant back pain from the surgery. As soon as she went back to sleep, I fell into Scott's arms and just cried.

I'm not sure if they were tears of joy because the surgery was over, or because she was not paralyzed. Were the tears because I knew that she would no longer suffer with back pain? Were they just tears from all the stress and anxiety that had built up during the 10 hours of waiting for her to return from surgery?

After that long and exhausting day, Scott went home while I stayed with Morgan in the ICU. Hospital regulations were that only one parent could stay with the child. Believe me as a parent, you do not get any rest or sleep in the ICU.

If it's not your child's machines going off, it's the patient in the next room. I heard machines beeping and nurses rushing to attend to the sounds. I desperately needed some sleep, the day was too much for me to bear, but I wouldn't be anywhere other than right beside my daughter. I needed to watch over her and make sure that everything was ok.

Morgan's spine was fused from T4 – T11, the T part refers to the thoracic part of the spine, meaning the upper to middle part of the back.

The spine is divided into 4 sections, the neck is the cervical spine, and it goes from C1 – C8.

The thoracic spine goes from T1 – T12, the lumbar spine, which is the area of the back that most people complain of having pain, goes from L1 – L5.

The real lower part of the spine is the sacral which goes from S1 – S4. So basically, she had just over 66% of her upper spine fused together.

The next day was amazing. Morgan was so excited that the surgery was over and insisted on calling her grade 6 teacher. Her teacher had been so supportive of Morgan while she was going through this difficult time pre-surgery. I know it meant a lot to Morgan to speak with her.

Unfortunately, cell phones didn't work in the ICU and Morgan was stuck in her bed, hooked up to all these machines. The nurses in the ICU unit removed many of these machines and attached a few others to the bed while they wheeled her to a desk phone. The teacher was as surprised as the nurses were that Morgan was comfortable enough to call.

That day, Morgan was moved into a regular room and over the next few days she was so happy to have so many friends visit her. She did have quite a bit of pain from the surgery, but she was handling it like a trooper.

Morgan was out of the hospital and at home in record time. It was so nice to be back home and selfishly to be back in my own bed, but there were also concerns. When we were in the hospital if something seemed awry, we could always check with the nurse, at home, I was the nurse.

The power of youth always amazed me. Morgan was so excited for surgery to be over with and so happy to be home, she just wanted her life to return to normal.

She reminded me of what the orthopaedic surgeon had told her before surgery. "Once you have surgery, it will be as if you never had scoliosis!" I wanted to appreciate those words, but I still had not recovered from that 10-hour stint in the hospital waiting area.

At this point, we were feeling good. She seemed to be recovering well. Yet, our journey was far from over.

SIXTEEN

PAIN GIRL

The first post surgical visit to the orthopaedic unit was upon us and Morgan was so excited to meet up with the surgeon and nurse number two, as well as spend some time with the psychologist, all of whom had visited Morgan while she had been in the ICU.

The doctor told Morgan that she did a fantastic job recovering from surgery and that the x-ray was clear and showed that everything was coming along as expected.

He did tell us that because Morgan now had metal rods in her spine this would cause some difficulty in getting an accurate picture of her spine. Morgan was beaming, she was proud of herself, and I was so proud of her and so happy that the worst was behind us.

Her curve pre-surgery had been at 62 degrees, it took 10 months for her to have surgery and the curve had increased 2 degrees a month. I tried to put that all behind us. When I saw Morgan smiling, knowing that she would no longer have back pain, that she could return to normalcy once the healing process was over made it all okay.

The surgeon told Morgan that there was a 6 – 12-month healing period, at which time, she could not lift heavy things, could not run and or participate in any sport, so gym class was out of the question.

Summer 2007 was extremely long. Many of Morgan's friends could not visit as their parents did not want them to encourage Morgan to do anything that could hinder the healing process.

I wished those parents would have called me so I could have told them to have their child come visit to just sit and talk, sit in the hot tub or watch a movie together. Morgan needed to have her friends around and they simply weren't because of fear or misunderstanding.

The highlight of the summer was when the psychologist from the orthopedic unit called to say that there was an art therapy program for children who had undergone major surgery or had a major illness. Morgan enjoyed this art therapy camp and it seemed to help her to see that she was not the only young person who had to deal with a major surgery or a serious health issue.

Just before school started, Morgan had a scheduled appointment with the surgeon once more. Morgan had mentioned that she was having some upper back pain once again and the surgeon told her that it was quite normal to still feel some pain but that within a few months everything would be fine again.

Grade seven started off on the wrong foot for Morgan. I knew that she was having difficulty in school mainly because every teacher would chastise her if they saw her running down the hallway like the other children were.

While I could appreciate that they were doing this for her own benefit, at the age of 12, it was too difficult for Morgan to see the positive side of the teachers' restrictions.

Moreover, she had to have gym class every day, a whole hour was dedicated to gym, and she could not participate. Although I had requested that Morgan be permitted to remain in the library or get extra help with her math. It was clear that she needed extra help in this area, she was forced to sit on the bench and watch all the other children play sports.

Did the school have to make it out to be a punishment for her? She could not participate in physical education class through no fault of her own. Yet, they made her sit there day after day while she watched other children enjoying themselves. This served as a constant reminder that she was different from them, that she was not a "normal" kid.

Six months post operation, the surgeon gave Morgan the green light to go ahead and participate in gym class. Morgan mentioned to the surgeon that her upper back was still in pain. He reassured us that the pain was normal and that the x-ray showed that her surgery had healed nicely, and she was free to be a 12-year-old.

There were many high fives in our house that evening. All three of us were excited that the surgery was a success and that we could all carry on with our lives. Amazing, just amazing that all of this was now behind us.

Before spring break in 2008 Morgan did copious amounts of research and discovered a package to Cuba. She did a whole presentation to Scott and I showing us how "cheap" this trip really was.

We had been to Mexico a few months prior, but we had never been to Cuba. Scott and I were impressed with the work she had done to put this presentation together. We decided to go ahead and book a spring break trip to Cuba. Scott couldn't come as we had just had a vacation and he needed to be at work. It was just going to be the two of us.

It was during this trip that I became seriously concerned about Morgan's upper back and the pain that she was experiencing. The surgeon had said to "just give it time", but this didn't seem right to me.

Here we are in a beautiful destination with incredible weather, yet Morgan said she couldn't walk up and down the beach. I encouraged her to take small walks on the beach so that she could wiggle her toes in the white sand. There wasn't any white sand in Calgary.

When we returned from our vacation in Cuba, I booked another appointment with the surgeon. The office arranged for Morgan to have both an x-ray and a scan. Sure enough, just as the surgeon had said before, everything was perfectly fine with Morgan's spine.

I asked the surgeon and the nurse what we were supposed to do as this pain was now interfering with Morgan's sleep and even her schoolwork. We were told to return to Morgan's paediatrician as perhaps her back wasn't completely healed, and he could prescribe some mild pain relief for her.

We are now one year post surgery and the surgeon had told us that at most the healing process would be one year. How are they just shifting the responsibility to Dr. Wong?

They obviously did not believe her. I could tell by the way they spoke to her and tried to make her believe that the pain was not real.

I know my daughter; this pain is real. In fact, I believe that Morgan has a higher pain tolerance than the average child. Morgan is not just making up the pain to skip school, in fact, she never wants to miss school even if she hasn't had enough sleep. What a true warrior.

Thankfully Dr. Wong was back, it was so nice just to have him around to speak with, he was always so reassuring. He reviewed the x-ray and the scan and said that he couldn't see anything wrong either.

The difference here is that he believed Morgan, he knew that Morgan was experiencing pain and he was compassionate and made Morgan feel that he was behind her, not fighting her.

After a few months of the mild pain medication that Dr. Wong had prescribed, I lost it, seriously lost it. Morgan had been awake for most of the night. I knew because I was right there with her trying to comfort her, trying to reassure her that everything was going to be ok. How was everything going to be ok. I had no clue. I just had to reassure her.

I contacted the nurse in the orthopedic unit, and I wasn't happy. I didn't have much sleep the night before, but Morgan was finally sleeping. I wasn't going to wake her up for school. We had to get to the bottom of this. It was going on for too long and Morgan couldn't function. I couldn't even bear to imagine the pain that she was in.

I explained to the nurse everything that Morgan had gone through over the past few months and how the medication prescribed by Dr. Wong wasn't working. I beschouwed the point where Morgan was not sleeping at all, and that the previous night was the icing on the cake and that something needed to be done.

The nurse was clearly taken aback by my words and her tone of voice said that she didn't care, she responded "**There is nothing wrong with your daughter!**"

Later that afternoon, the orthopedic nurse contacted me saying that she had set up an appointment for Morgan to meet with the psychologist in the orthopedic unit to see if they couldn't get to the bottom of things, still implying that this pain was not real, and that Morgan was faking it.

At this point, I was thinking that this was just a brush off. I knew that I had to keep going forward and hopefully keep Morgan positive about the fact that something was being done about her back pain. In reality, nothing was being done.

Maybe something good did come out of the meeting with the orthopedic psychologist, as she referred Morgan to the paediatric pain clinic. Morgan was having such difficulty dealing with this pain and as her mother it was killing me. I want to scream to the universe, or perhaps to anyone who would listen. "PLEASE HELP MY DAUGHTER".

We met with the paediatric pain doctor and instantly felt a connection. She seemed to be so sympathetic to Morgan's pain and seemed to want to help. She seemed like an ally, like she was someone we could rely on.

Oh, how the tables turned after a couple of appointments. Without us being made aware, the orthopaedic nurse joined us for one of the appointments. She made it very clear that there was absolutely nothing wrong with Morgan's back and that Morgan was imagining the pain.

I wasn't backing down. I knew that Morgan was not making up the pain. I knew that she was in horrific pain. No one was helping, no one in the medical field believed her except for Dr. Wong of course.

Dr. Wong mentioned that if the pain got too severe that we should head to the emergency room. We had gone to the emergency room a time or two before, but this one evening when the pain was particularly bad, we did exactly as Dr. Wong had suggested, and went to the emergency room. We were greeted by the triage nurse who immediately laughed with her colleagues and said, "**Oh look, it's 'pain girl'.**"

I couldn't believe my ears, here we were in a place that everyone assumes is professional and has our children's mental and physical health as a top priority and they can be this rude and callous?

It was a very difficult balance as a mother to know what to do in a situation like that. You want to defend your child, yet you want to teach your child to ignore such nonsense.

I wanted to scream. I felt like slapping the nurse and using vulgar language. Yet, I wanted to teach Morgan not to react in these ways or resort to violence.

I chose to ignore the comments as difficult as it was. I wasn't sure that Morgan had heard them, and I didn't want to draw more attention to the stupidity than need be.

We waited for hours with Morgan in agonizing pain. We finally met with a lovely doctor who gave Morgan a shot of morphine and suggested that we continue our journey with the orthopedic unit and the pain clinic.

I explained to this lovely young man that we tried, desperately tried, to get either one of those places to understand and to help Morgan. She slept on the way home. One of the most peaceful sleeps I had seen her have in a long while.

Over the next week we discovered that Morgan's orthopedic surgeon was leaving the Calgary area and heading out east. The only way this was discovered is when I called the orthopedic unit to book an appointment for Morgan.

The pain was intolerable at this point, and something had to be done. The nurse told me that there was nothing wrong with Morgan's spine, and that she was faking the pain. She continued and said that if I thought that Morgan needed to see an orthopedic surgeon that Dr. Wong could refer her back to the orthopaedic unit and she would be put on the list and be seen in two to three years. This is Canada, how could this be possible?

I hung up the phone and just cried. What was I going to do? What was I going to tell Morgan? Once again, the healthcare system made me feel like a failure. Was I a failure? Why did we have to fight so hard for basic care? Why did we have to live life like this? Why do families have to suffer so much?

Oddly enough, shortly after my phone conversation with the orthopedic nurse, the psychologist from the unit called to say that since Morgan was already 18 months post surgery, she wasn't entitled to additional sessions with the psychologist.

What, like seriously? The psychologist was the most beneficial part of the journey for Morgan as we fought our way through this system. I begged her to keep Morgan on.

I asked if she could not make an exception and keep Morgan on because of the pain that she was having. Morgan always listened intently and repeated the pain management lessons that she had learnt from this woman.

"Please" I begged, "Morgan needs your guidance more than ever", and just like that she told me she had to go and hung up.

When Morgan returned home from school, I couldn't tell her that I had spoken with either of these people. I didn't really know what to say, or how I was going to say it. I needed to discuss everything with Scott.

I needed him to know that even begging for help wasn't working. I was reduced to begging, it was for my daughter, so it was not beneath me. But no one seemed to care or listen.

SEVENTEEN

DAD'S FED UP

Scott and I discussed selling everything we owned in Calgary and putting the money towards taking Morgan to the United States for treatment. We had done quite a bit of research and felt confident that she would be taken seriously at many of the phenomenal medical institutions in the States.

It was hard to digest that we were even considering going to the United States for treatment, but we felt as if we had exhausted all avenues. Morgan's spinal fusion surgery was 18 months ago, and she still was in debilitating pain.

I booked an appointment to meet up with Dr. Wong to get all of Morgan's medical records. He could see the desperation in my eyes, and he knew that we felt that there was no other way to ensure that Morgan got the medical care that she needed. In his usual fashion, Dr. Wong made me feel as if I were doing the right thing. He had always told me "Mother's know."

Dr. Wong asked me if we would consider the Orthopaedic Hospital in Montreal as an alternative to going to the United States. We never thought of the Orthopaedic Hospital in Montreal as being a viable alternative. It seemed so far away. We knew that there were many places in the United States that were physically closer to us in Calgary.

Dr. Wong had contacted a representative of the Orthopaedic Hospital in Montreal and just like that the ball was in motion.

Yes indeed, with Dr. Wong's help, we would be heading to Montreal to meet with Dr. Oliver in the Spring of 2009.

We still had an appointment with the paediatric pain clinic in Calgary and both Scott and I knew that the doctor would also say that her time with Morgan had to come to an end as nothing was wrong. We kept the appointment, however instead of Morgan meeting up with the doctor, Scott and I showed up.

The pain clinic doctor herself seemed so nice and seemed to have a genuine concern about the pain that Morgan was in; however, it appeared as if she was greatly influenced or bullied into believing what the orthopaedic nurse was telling her.

Now that I knew that we had this appointment booked to meet an orthopaedic surgeon in Montreal, I felt more brazen.

I had a newfound confidence that allowed me to feel as if I didn't have to take their bull shit anymore. I knew that something was wrong with Morgan and everyone, starting with the orthopaedic surgeon that performed her surgery, the orthopaedic nurse, the orthopaedic psychologist and even the paediatric pain clinic doctor would not change my mind. Thankfully, Dr. Wong was and always had been on our side.

The shock on the pain doctor's face was very noticeable when she saw Scott walk into the room, she had expected to see Morgan. We were surrounded by everyone who had worked with Morgan except for the surgeon himself.

We had the nurse, the psychologist and the pain doctor. I assume that they thought that they would have a united front to let Morgan know that "Pain Girl" was faking it.

Scott was amazing as he addressed these individuals. Sadly, to say that even today, when a man says something, it seems to hold more value than if a woman says the exact same thing. I had been advocating for Morgan for months trying to get everyone to see that she was in horrendous pain, yet they seemed to listen more attentively to Scott.

The pain doctor was first to speak, and it was obvious that she felt quite uneasy. She had never met Scott and was relying on the information from the orthopaedic nurse and now she would have to explain herself to him. She was careful with her words, she looked up at both the nurse and the psychologist to ensure that they had her back, no pun intended.

Scoliosis Does Not Hurt

She told Scott that all tests pointed to the fact that there was nothing wrong with Morgan's back, and after much discussion, it was evident that indeed nothing was wrong with Morgan, and we needed to understand that it was quite likely that Morgan was faking it for attention.

The nurse cut in and was proud to say that both the x-ray and the scan showed that nothing was wrong with Morgan's back and that the fusion was a success. When Scott pointed out that the surgeon had told us that it would be difficult to read an x-ray and a scan due to the fact that she had hardware in her back, the nurse just shook her head.

Scott continued to explain that Morgan was awake most nights in severe pain, and if she were "faking it" as they had felt she was, she would most probably want to be skipping school. In fact, Morgan insisted on going to school, even the days that we had felt that she should stay at home due to pain and/or lack of sleep, she did not want to miss even one day of school.

Scott asked all three of these ladies, if that made sense, that a young girl would be faking pain yet continue to go to school everyday. He continued by saying, if I were faking pain, I would be using this as an excuse to not go to work.

He said that he couldn't understand why they thought she was faking it and pushing through the pain to go to school every day. What was her objective?

Not one of these three individuals had a response, they were dumbfounded, they weren't prepared for a meeting with the father of this young girl complaining of excruciating pain. They were ready to bully this young child, to make her feel that she was imagining this pain and that she had to stop complaining because it was falling on deaf ears.

I could feel my blood boil, every time that they spoke and implied that nothing was wrong with Morgan and that it was all in her head. It was more than I could take. Scott was doing an excellent job, but he hadn't been part of the entire process. Sure, I had discussed everything with him, but he was not at every appointment, he was not the person who listened to these so-called professionals badger Morgan.

I still couldn't believe that this was the best they would do. Not could do but would do. They wanted to be done and they seemed to care very little that we were talking about a child. A child that was in such pain she could barely function. They found this amusing. How could this even be happening?

Morgan and I flew out to Montreal in the spring or 2009 to meet with Dr. Oliver. Morgan had done her own research and felt confident that Dr. Oliver would be in a position to help her. I tried not to get too hopeful, but I was desperate. I knew something was wrong, but would Dr. Oliver believe Morgan? It was so difficult for me to wrap my head around things, the original surgeon did not believe her, the orthopaedic nurse did not believe her, the psychologist in the orthopaedic unit did not believe her and the paediatric pain clinic did not believe her, so here we are on a plane to Montreal desperately hoping that Dr. Oliver would believe her.

Both Morgan and I were extremely nervous to meet with Dr. Oliver after the experience we had had in Calgary, but we had to try. Dr. Wong had confidence in the Orthopaedic Hospital, we had to go with that, as I had confidence in Dr. Wong.

We met with Dr. Oliver, and he seemed so patient and kind, he made us feel comfortable, as comfortable as Dr. Wong had over the years. Dr. Oliver said the exact same thing that both the x-ray and scan showed that everything was perfect, but he believed Morgan, he knew that something was wrong. He said that occasionally the rods and screws from the original spinal fusion had to be removed.

That is all we needed, was for a doctor to believe Morgan. Whatever was wrong was wrong and he would remove the hardware and Morgan would be fine. He stated that without a doubt, two years after spinal fusion a spine would be fully fused, and hardware was no longer required. Her surgery to remove her hardware was scheduled for June 3, 2009.

Scoliosis Does Not Hurt

The relief that all three of us felt was indescribable. Finally, an orthopaedic surgeon believed Morgan, and something was going to be done about it.

June 3, 2009, was here and Morgan was about to have her second spine surgery, this time it was at the Orthopaedic Hospital in Montreal. Without a doubt, here we were halfway across the country and sitting in a waiting room waiting for our daughter to come out of surgery. It felt different this time, I'm not sure why, could it be because Dr. Oliver believed Morgan, could it be because we fought so hard to get to this point that we were prepared for the agonizing wait in the surgical waiting room?

Dr Oliver met with Scott and I immediately following the surgery to let us know that as far as he could see everything was perfectly fine, he removed the hardware, and felt that things should go back to normal for Morgan. I remembered how after her first surgery, no one came to meet us, no one reassured us that everything was fine. We only found out that she was in the ICU unit because of an announcement on the loudspeaker. Certainly, having Dr. Oliver meeting with us after the surgery gave us a level of confidence.

He implied that he thought perhaps the hardware had been irritating Morgan's back but now that the hardware was out, she shouldn't have anymore pain.

I was so relieved to see her after her surgery and happy to tell her that Dr. Oliver said that everything was fine and that she wouldn't have anymore pain. It was such a relief.

As with hospital policy Scott returned to the hotel room and I stayed with Morgan. As I watched her sleep, tears rolled down my face, I whispered to her "It's over love, all the pain is over."

She was eager to get back to school and to live a pain free life. She often referred to the quote from the original surgeon, "Once you recover from the spinal fusion surgery, it will be as if you never had scoliosis at all." She clung to this statement and desperately wanted it to be true.

Once back at school, Morgan felt worse pain than before. Could this be possible? How could it be possible? Now that we were more aware of what scoliosis is and what body changes to look for, it appeared as if her curve was increasing.

Impossible! She had her spinal fusion in May of 2007, we were now in September of 2009, sure the rods were removed in June 2009, but just as both spinal surgeons had said, at most it would take one year for her spine to fuse, and technically after this one-year period, she would not need the rods.

Between the pain and what appeared to be an increasing curve, we contacted the hospital in Montreal, and they ordered an emergency x-ray and C.T. scan. As unbelievable as it sounds Morgan's back did not fully fuse from the original surgery, she had pseudoarthrosis.

Pseudoarthrosis is a medical term used to describe a lack of fusion, meaning that the spinal fusion was not completed. Medical experts feel that for most patients, motion in the area that is not fused can cause pain like that of a broken bone that never heals.

Looking online at various sites I discovered that it is expected that after undergoing a spinal fusion the individual may find relief of their pre-surgical and surgical pain within three months of the surgery, but afterwards they should be symptom free.

It is evident that once the patient is beyond their postsurgical restrictions period and are returning to normal activity, if they still are complaining of pain, even worse pain than what they started with, it would be understandable that the surgeon would consider pseudoarthrosis.

As I am reviewing site after site, I am overwhelmed with what I am reading. It's as if Morgan was walking around with a broken spine. Keeping in mind that the original surgery was in May 2007, and we are now in September 2009. How barbaric of any medical system to think that this was ok for a child?

I tried to understand what Morgan was going through. I can't even imagine how painful and frustrating this has all been for her when all the doctors, surgeons and nurses implied that she was faking.

I am beyond upset, there are no words that could explain my emotions because what could I do? Absolutely nothing, for over 2 years my daughter has been walking around with a broken spine and although I tried to get her the help she needed, I was not successful.

Who should I call? Who should I write to? I have gone the government route to no avail. I tried the emergency room route, but nothing. I tried the pediatric pain clinic to no avail. The orthopaedic psychologist blew me off. The orthopaedic nurse was condescending and rude. The orthopedic surgeon insisted that she was fine. I tried and tried, yet it wasn't enough. The guilt was overwhelming, yet I knew that there was nothing more that I could have done. As a parent you want to take away your child's pain, this is very normal and very understandable, I felt like a failure. I could not take away her pain, I hope that she realizes later in life that I tried everything that I could to take away this horrific pain.

I tried not to relive the countless nights where Morgan tried to fall asleep with a horrible burning pain in her upper back. I tried not to relive the times my daughter asked me why they didn't believe her.

I tried not to focus on the things I could not change. Yet, I am human, and this is my daughter, my only child. My whole-body hurts with the knowledge of the pain that she must have endured over these past two years.

As only Morgan could, she carried on. The strength of this child never ceased to amaze me. She was fine with the fact that she would require a third spinal surgery and a second spinal fusion. She just wanted to be pain free. She just wanted the words of her original orthopedic surgeon to be true. "Once you have the surgery, it will be as if you never had scoliosis at all."

Due to the fact that Morgan's spine was not fully fused from the original fusion in May of 2007, we had to have another surgery to re-fuse the part of the spine that did not fuse. The surgery at the Orthopaedic Hospital in Montreal was scheduled for December 2009.

Out of the blue that December, Scott got sick, really sick. Scott rarely was sick, but he had been home for a few days and had been complaining of pain in his rib area, the pain was so intense that it made it difficult for him to speak. He thought that the pain might be due to a hit he took in hockey.

Yes, that does sound truly Canadian. However, this hockey injury was not getting any better, in fact Scott could hardly get out of bed. I was finally able to convince him to get to the emergency room where he was diagnosed with pneumonia. He apparently waited too long, and the pneumonia had settled in.

Scott was admitted to the hospital, and I knew that this was serious. I was so very worried about him in the hospital, but the worry got worse, because I now had a choice,

I could stay with Scott in the hospital in Calgary or fly out to Montreal with Morgan while she endures her third spine surgery. We did think that we might have been able to postpone Morgan's surgery, but both Scoot and I knew of the pain that Morgan was in and we could not in good conscience allow the surgery to be postponed.

Of course, there was no thought to it, both Scott and I knew that I had to be in Montreal with Morgan.

As Morgan and I flew out to Montreal, I felt horrible for leaving Scott in the hospital on his own. I so wanted to be there with him while he was going through this health crisis, but I had to be with Morgan, there was no question about that. Throughout the flight to Montreal, I fretted about how Scott was doing in Calgary, and I was so very worried about him recovering from the pneumonia, I knew that he had waited too long.

Surgery date was upon us and I said good- bye to Morgan as she headed into surgery, my thoughts were on how Scott was doing in the Calgary hospital.

Seriously, my husband was in a Calgary hospital and not doing too well with pneumonia and my daughter was in a hospital in Montreal about to have her back sliced into for the third time.

I cried and cried and cried. I was allowed to; it was all too much for me to handle. I was alone, trapped with my thoughts. Was Scott going to make it, was Morgan going to make it, would I lose both of them on the same day in different cities?

I tried to turn my attention to other more positive thoughts. Christmas would soon be upon us. Morgan would finally be out of pain and Scott would be doing well and all three of us would be celebrating Christmas together in our little home in the Calgary suburb of Lakeview.

Believe me I tried. I desperately tried not to think on the negative side. My gut instinct told me that I must think of only positive thoughts, but it could happen, I could lose both of them on the same day and poof just like that my life would be turned upside down.

Thankfully, the surgery is over, and Morgan returns to her room and the first thing she asks is how her dad is doing in Calgary.

Here she is having gone through a horrific surgery and she is more concerned about her dad than herself. We called Scott on his cell phone, not sure if he would be able to answer or not, he was anxiously awaiting our call, he was weak, but he said that he was doing better.

So much relief, my daughter had awakened from surgery and seemed to be doing fine and my husband was alright in a hospital so far away.

During this spinal fusion surgery Morgan's spine was fused one additional vertebra at the top and one below her original fusion. The original spinal fusion was from T4 – T11, this new fusion was from T3 – T12.

I tried to let myself relax a little. Would this nightmare finally be over? Or would there be more obstacles waiting for us?

EIGHTEEN

DRAMA QUEEN

In early 2010, Morgan had an appointment at the paediatric rheumatology clinic in Calgary shortly after her third spine surgery. Dr. Wong had referred Morgan to the rheumatology clinic as she also suffered with generalized joint pain and discomfort.

The orthopaedic clinic and the rheumatology clinic were side by side and when we were heading to the rheumatologist office, we bumped into the nurse from the orthopaedic unit. Morgan, being a regular 14-year-old ran up to the nurse and said, "You know what, I did have a problem with my spine after my spinal fusion, my spine wasn't fully fused. I had pseudoarthrosis. There really was an issue with my spine."

Just from the sound of her voice you could tell that Morgan was excited to let this nurse know that indeed there was an issue. She wanted to share the good news with the nurse that her spine was once again fused.

Only a child could be that optimistic. As for myself, I didn't even want to look at that woman. I remembered clearly her tone and the abrasive way in which she told me that nothing was wrong with my daughter and that I could have had Dr. Wong refer her to the orthopaedic unit and that she would have been seen in two to three years. The thought of having my daughter live with that horrific pain for another two to three years was gut wrenching.

She looked directly at Morgan and simply said "How did we know Morgan, you are such a drama queen!" Of course, she ran into the protective custody behind the doors of the orthopaedic unit.

Really, what could I have said? What could I have said in front of my daughter? There is such a fine line, and did it really matter? I thought about sending a letter to the orthopaedic unit but seriously? Had I not tried that approach before by contacting my MLA? Did it really work? Obviously not, and that's why we had to head out to the Orthopaedic Hospital in Montreal.

A few weeks later, Scott and Morgan had seen an episode on Mystery Diagnosis and felt that the lady portrayed in the episode mirrored Morgan in many ways. After discussion of this episode with Dr. Wong, he referred us to a genetic specialist, to check out things and to get his opinion.

We certainly kept fighting, we knew we had to keep fighting to try to determine why Morgan was going through everything that she was going through and to understand what lied ahead for her.

In February 2010, we met with this genetic specialist in the southwest community of Discovery Ridge and to our surprise, he indicated that indeed Morgan did have Ehlers-Danlos Syndrome. He explained to us that Ehlers-Danlos Syndrome, more commonly referred to as EDS, is a hereditary disorder of connective tissue.

The episode of Mystery Diagnosis that Scott and Morgan had watched was about a woman who lived with Ehlers Danlos syndrome.

The doctor explained that there are many proteins in connective tissue and one of the key proteins is collagen. With EDS, there are faults in the genes that determine how the body makes collagen. This leads to the connective tissue becoming weaker.

Of course, most of this was going over our heads. Morgan and I just stared at each other. Incredibly, just as she had known that she had scoliosis before being tested, she knew she had EDS before anyone had any clue.

The genetic specialist was thorough, he reviewed everything about Morgan, from her birth to her walking and speech. We reviewed the issues with her motor skills, learning disability, scoliosis and of course pseudoarthrosis.

He continued that with the hypermobility type of EDS that there is joint hypermobility and joint instability, injury and pain in most joints and muscles.

He was such an accommodating doctor and he agreed that the EDS could be the reason that Morgan had difficulty crawling and learning to walk due to the instability that she felt. Quite possibly it was the reason that her speech was delayed and without a doubt it is the reason behind her scoliosis and pseudoarthrosis.

Armed with this information, I didn't know if I were happy that we finally had a name that we could definitely say was the cause of everything Morgan had gone through. Or was I angry because I tried so desperately to find out for years!

I didn't know if this changed anything. For years, I was focused on finding out what was wrong with Morgan? What did Morgan have? What were we missing? Did it matter? Morgan was still Morgan, and we still had a mountain to climb.

According to the Ehlers-Danlos Society web page:

" Connective tissue is everywhere in the body. It provides support and structure to other tissues and organs including bone, ligaments, tendons, blood vessels, lymphatic vessels, the tissue that holds the gastrointestinal tract in place, etc.

There are many proteins in connective tissue. One of the key proteins is collagen. In the Ehlers-Danlos syndromes, there are faults in the genes that determine how the body makes collagen, and/or in some subtypes other proteins that work alongside collagen. This leads to the connective tissue becoming weaker. Different tissues and organs can be affected in diverse ways depending on the genetic fault. This explains why there are several subtypes of EDS."[5]

As the months progressed, Morgan still had a lot of pain despite thinking that it should be otherwise. It was as if we were living in a nightmare, how could this be? How come my daughter

---

[5] https://www.ehlers-danlos.com

continued to suffer? Why couldn't this be over? When will this be over?

By spring 2010 I contacted the Orthopaedic Hospital in Montreal to let them know about the situation. Morgan was still experiencing upper back pain and it was debilitating. The surgeon recommended that we wait a few more months to see if the pain would subside.

This was easy for him to say, but Morgan's original surgery was in 2007, we were now in 2010 and she had already had three spinal surgeries. We lived a nightmare throughout this whole time, we need the pain to end. She needs to return to a normal life. Whatever happened to that promise her original surgeon had made, "Once the surgery is over, it will be as if you never had scoliosis at all." Of course, we can't forget the original comments of efficient nurse number 1 in the orthopaedic unit "Scoliosis Does Not Hurt."

In August 2010, we were headed back to the Orthopaedic Hospital in Montreal for x-rays and CT scans. Morgan and I were waiting anxiously in the examining room for Dr. Oliver to let us know the results. I didn't want to think of what could be wrong, is it pseudoarthrosis again? Are they going to be able to tell that it is indeed pseudoarthrosis, they couldn't tell the last time apparently because of the hardware in her back? Now we were aware of the diagnosis of EDS.

Dr. Oliver came in and with his magnetic smile, he brightened the whole room. We discussed our meeting with the genetic specialist in Calgary and his diagnosis of EDS. He was always upbeat and positive, and it was very much appreciated.

He said that he couldn't see anything wrong with Morgan's spine and he is confident that all of her vertebrae from $T_3 - T_{12}$ are fused. He suggested that we speak with a pain management doctor in Montreal.

We met with the Montreal pain management doctor, and he gave us a referral form for Morgan to meet with one of his students that was now practising in Calgary. He felt that it would be much better for Morgan to meet with a Calgary pain specialist as that is where we lived.

Morgan was disappointed and fearful that she would end up in the same loop as she had after her first spinal fusion. I assured her that if the pain management doctor in Montreal was referring her directly to a pain specialist in Calgary that she would be seen quickly. I was confident of this, perhaps a little too confident.

As soon as we got back home to Calgary, I phoned the pain clinic and explained the whole story to the receptionist and asked where she would like me to fax the referral to. I can only assume that the young lady who answered the phone was having a bad day, as she was so rude to me. "Well normally doctor's fax us the request directly!"

I thought to myself, did she not hear a word I just said? I told her about meeting with the professor of the pain clinic doctor who, he assured us, would take care of Morgan. Like seriously, who cares if I fax the referral to them or if it came from the doctor's office from Montreal?

I had to continue being patient. If I have learnt one thing while going through this crazy health care maze with my daughter it's that the people making the appointments are critical to actually getting an appointment, they are the gatekeepers.

As patiently as I could I re-explained that the Montreal pain clinic doctor had taught the doctor in Montreal and felt confident that he would be able to help Morgan. I was losing my patience, but I knew I had to keep this woman talking if I wanted a chance of having Morgan visit this specialist.

"Who does this Montreal pain doctor think he is?" she asks aggressively. I know that she is seriously irritated by now. Why? I have no idea. I am all peaches and cream nice to her and I am trying my best to get this woman to book an appointment for Morgan.

I did not want to irritate this woman anymore than I had to. I then asked her if she could have the doctor call me himself. I am certain that she felt as if I was going over her head. She screamed at me saying that the pain clinic in Calgary was busy and the doctor in Montreal had no business in misleading us.

I explain that I would still like to fax the referral to the pain clinic and wait to hear from the doctor himself. She hesitantly agreed but indicated that she needed to ask a few basic questions first, like my daughter's name, address, phone number and date of birth.

When I provided her with Morgan's date of birth she erupted in severe anger, as if I had just hit her on the side of her head. She continued, "Why are you calling here, this is an adult pain clinic, your daughter is only 15 years old?" I wanted to thank her for being so good at math and enlightening me on the age of my own child, but I knew better.

"Never heard of it, not possible, never happens here, will not happen here!" she continued as I pleaded with her to have the doctor contact me directly because the Montreal pain specialist felt confident that he could help her.

I was shaking as I got off the phone. I felt like I was failing Morgan once again. I was trying, really trying but I felt defeated.

How was I going to tell Morgan about my conversation with the pain clinic in Calgary? She would be so disappointed and feel like once again, her pain was going to be ignored by the medical community.

September 2010 and Morgan is excited to start a new adventure, she is switching from private school into public school. This was her decision and although we were now more comfortable with her being in private school, we understood that she wanted to attend a more standardized school setting.

In grade 10, gym was mandatory and while I was nervous about Morgan participating in gym class, she was not. I had to let go. I had to let Morgan be her own person. She was 15 years old and needed to know and understand any possible limitations due to her scoliosis and EDS.

What could possibly go wrong in gym class?

NINETEEN

THE AMBULANCE IS ON ITS WAY

Mid-September 2010, I got a call from the school saying that Morgan had an accident during gym class and that an ambulance was on its way. My heart raced. I couldn't think straight. Yet, I drove to the school not really knowing how I got there. I called Scott to let him know what was going on. He said he would meet me there.

I had no clue which roads I took but I made it. I kept saying to myself that she should not be in gym class and why did the school make it mandatory for her to participate in gym? I couldn't even imagine what happened to her and why she needed an ambulance.

Both Scott and I saw the ambulance in the school parking lot. A paramedic came over and told us that it appeared that Morgan suffered a mild concussion from being cross checked by a fellow student. Morgan indicated that she was doing well. However, due to the concussion they felt that she needed to be taken to the hospital.

Another paramedic came over and chastised me for not providing all of Morgan's medical history to the school. They indicated that while she was unconscious, another student informed them that Morgan had spina bifida. Of course, that is not what she had. Did no one read the documents we were required to submit with her registration? It took me hours to complete these documents.

My heart was racing just to hear that she had been unconscious. I didn't want to waste any time explaining it to them. At the time that Morgan had registered at the school, I completed reams of paperwork outlining all of Morgan's health conditions and I never mentioned that she had spina bifida. Yes, she had an issue with her spine, but it wasn't spina bifida.

Thankfully, all Morgan had was a minor concussion and I was assured that the accident at school had not impacted her spine at all. At this point I have no idea what is or is not true. Could I really trust what any healthcare professional told me? I still did not want Morgan to participate in gym class, but that wasn't going to change anything.

The following day, I made sure to speak with the school secretary about Morgan's medical information not being available to the paramedics. She told me that due to the fact that Morgan was a new student they hadn't had enough time to input the information. She assured me that she did have the information on paper and would input it immediately.

And wouldn't you know it, late October and I got another call from the school this time telling me that I had better rush to the hospital as Morgan was on her way there via ambulance, the secretary calling had no additional information.

By the time she hung up, I was having trouble breathing, my panic mode was full on. I knew I had to calm down if I expected Scott to understand me on the phone.

I couldn't reach Scott on the phone, so I left to the emergency room without him being aware of things. I knew that I had to determine what was wrong before leaving him a panicked message.

It took fifteen minutes to drive there, yet it felt like hours. I kept wondering what had happened to Morgan. Not knowing what was wrong, my mind went to different places, none of them good.

I got to the hospital, and there I was by Morgan's side. She was lying on a stretcher in her torn sweatpants with a neck brace on. I tried not to project my worry and stress onto her, but this wasn't easy.

Sure enough, it was gym class again; she had fallen off a six-foot stage and landed on her neck. Apparently, she let out a loud scream, thankfully, the teacher was able to immobilize her and have someone call for the ambulance.

While the paramedics were briefing me on what happened. They told me that they were surprised that the school had no medical information about Morgan. I am beyond frustrated; it is now late October, and the school still claims not to have Morgan's medical information. How could this have happened again?

After x-rays and scans, it was determined that Morgan had injured her neck, but not too seriously. They also felt that she had a mild concussion once again.

I hated to sound like a broken record, but I was so concerned about her spine. While the neck is considered part of the spine, being the cervical spine. I was more concerned about the part of her spine that had been fused, which was basically all of her thoracic spine. Once again, I am assured that there was no impact to her thoracic spine, but could I believe them?

January 2011 was upon us and the weather in Calgary was brutal. Morgan was feeling more pain and discomfort in her spine but also in many of her joints. The genetic specialist had mentioned to us that the change in weather would be difficult for Morgan's joints. Whether from cold to hot or from hot to cold, it was the change and her ability to cope with the changes in temperatures.

Morgan was quite excited to learn that she would be speaking at a dinner to raise money for scoliosis research. She wanted to do something to make people more aware of the condition and how it affected those that suffered from it.

The Oilympics Hockey Tournament was in March 2011. Every year these fine men and women working in Calgary's oil and gas industry came together to compete in a hockey tournament. Scott had been part of this tradition year after year and always enjoyed participating and contributing to the charities that were selected by the Oilympics committee.

After many meetings, emails and phone calls the committee had agreed that there would be two charities this year with the main one being scoliosis research at the Orthopaedic Hospital in Montreal.

We all were so very happy that scoliosis research had been chosen, we had hoped to raise about $50,000 for the hospital's research foundation.

It was so especially important to me for Morgan to see that people were concerned about scoliosis. She was an avid participant in the Terry Fox run each year and often was the student that had collected the most money for cancer research.

When she was first diagnosed with scoliosis in August of 2006, we were out going door to door to collect money for the Terry Fox run, she had said in her 11-year-old voice, "How come people raise so much money for cancer research, yet no one raises any money for scoliosis research?"

I was so proud to let her know that because of her people were being made aware of scoliosis and its impact on so many children. I was so happy for her to see that everyone was at the dinner and auction to raise money for scoliosis research.

At the dinner, we were seated with Dr. Oliver, as well as representatives of the Orthopaedic Hospital from Montreal. Morgan found it quite different to be seated next to Dr. Oliver in a social setting rather than a hospital one.

After the delicious meal, Morgan and Dr. Oliver were about to speak about scoliosis, what it was, and what the Orthopaedic Hospital in Montreal does to help children that live with this debilitating condition.

Morgan nailed it; she was amazing. I cried as she described her ordeal. It was as if everything had sunk to the bottom and with each word, it came to the surface and it was real. Everything we had gone through was flashing through my mind as I listened to my daughter describe what she had endured.

I was very sad, but I was also very angry because a lot of what we had to go through didn't have to be that way.

Dr. Oliver gave an excellent talk about scoliosis and showed some samples of x-rays of some children who lived with the condition. He explained about the surgeries and most importantly spoke of how critical research into this condition was.

Scoliosis Does Not Hurt

It was almost like a fairy tale, none of us wanted the night to end. It was the feeling of doing something powerful to potentially help other children afflicted with scoliosis. It was so rewarding and put all of us on such an incredible high.

In April, a referral was made for Morgan to get a spinal injection to see if this would reduce or eliminate her pain. After much back and forth, believe me when I say much back and forth, Morgan was scheduled for her spinal injection.

Was I worried? Of course, I was. I didn't know what else to do to help my daughter with her pain. I had to keep fighting, that was my job. I am her mother, and I was determined to keep fighting.

After much discussion about being able to get spinal injections with hardware, Dr. Oliver stepped in to discuss the situation with the hospital in Calgary.

Morgan lived in extreme pain. This pain affected every aspect of her life, from school, to friends, to sleep, to happiness and to her overall mental health.

We entered the special services building in Calgary and Morgan was led away for the injection. I knew that Morgan was nervous. I doubted that she was as nervous as I was. I tried to portray a positive mind frame and hold on to hope that everything would be ok after this injection.

As I sat in the hallway where other patients are waiting for their injections or with a loved one. I can hear Morgan screaming. At first, I was so shocked. What about privacy?

I couldn't think or focus on anything. I just started crying, right there in the waiting area. I noticed a woman approaching me and she was trying to comfort me. I am not in the "comfort me" mindset, that was my daughter screaming in agony.

She had no clue what I'd been through and how dare she attempt to comfort me. Instead of lashing out, I let her know that I was ok. It obviously wasn't her fault that Morgan was in this situation.

As she took her seat, I noticed that she was talking with a younger gentleman who was obviously going through cancer treatment. I take note that we were in the special services building in the cancer centre.

I cried harder now, realizing that this woman was kind enough to try to comfort me while she was dealing with her son who was fighting cancer. I thought to myself, what a cruel world we live in, where children and young adults must suffer so much. Those were my thoughts at that moment. I felt defeated.

Thankfully, the needle was over, and we are on our way home. Morgan tells me that the needle was extremely painful and that she knows that it has not helped her one bit and is insistent that it will not help her.

I want to chastise her and tell her not to be so negative. If Dr. Oliver thought it would help, it would. But I know what she has been through. I know that she has developed a tough exterior where she doesn't want to believe a word any medical practitioner tells her. Could I blame her?

In July of 2011 we heard back from the Oilympic committee. They have a cheque that they want to present to the Orthopaedic Hospital in Montreal for scoliosis research. They made arrangements for us to meet with them at a restaurant just east of downtown in the quaint community of Inglewood.

While Dr. Oliver could not attend this luncheon on such short notice. A representative of the Orthopaedic Hospital was available for the luncheon and was presented with a cheque in the amount of $85,000.

We were amazed, we had hoped for $50,000, and this was well over what we had expected. All three of us were feeling quite proud that in Morgan's name the Orthopaedic Hospital had $85,000 for scoliosis research.

After discovering that the injection hadn't helped Morgan, Dr. Oliver arranged for us to go back to the Orthopaedic hospital in August 2011. At this point, he was unsure of how to help Morgan, but he promised that he would get to the bottom of the situation.

The days and nights at the hospital were long. Scott does not take the journey to Montreal with us, as we are unsure of how long we might be.

Scoliosis Does Not Hurt

For most of the day and evening we played cards and chatted, but Morgan can only focus on her back and wants the pain to be gone. She repeats what her original surgeon had told her "After surgery, it will be as if you never had scoliosis at all."

As her mother, I would do anything to take her pain. It was killing me to watch her suffer every day knowing that this has greatly impacted her life. She is a beautiful 16-year-old girl that just wants a normal life, was that too much to ask? I would rather endure this horrific pain I have witnessed over the past five years than to watch her go through it.

All I can do is be with her and wait. The waiting is hard but sadly, we are accustomed to it.

TWENTY

SPINE SURGERY NUMBER FOUR

Days turn into weeks and weeks turn into a month. We were at the Orthopaedic Hospital for about a month when Dr. Oliver said that he would put Morgan on an emergency surgical list, meaning that she possibly could have surgery at any hospital in Montreal.

The unfortunate part about being on this list is that Morgan could not eat anything all day and could only eat around 7 p.m. when they are sure that she will not have surgery that day.

This proved to be quite difficult for Morgan, but I stood with her. I promised her that I would not eat until she was able to. I must admit that every once in a while, when I told her that I was heading outside for some fresh air, I may have cheated a time or two. Even with the small cheats, I knew it was difficult not to eat anything until 7 p.m. This went on for a few days and Morgan was growing understandably impatient.

Finally, we were whisked off to the hospital where Morgan would have her surgery. To say that I was nervous would be an understatement. One would think that by now I was used to these long spine surgeries, but I was not.

While she was in surgery, I communicated with everyone back home in Calgary to let them know that she was having surgery. It was so difficult to be there without Scott, in fact the whole month was so long and trying.

This hospital set up was much different than what we were accustomed to. I felt like a professional waiting room critic by now. I was sitting right outside the doors from where she was having surgery. Thankfully, I couldn't hear a thing. I really didn't want to. I couldn't even begin to imagine how difficult it must be for her to have a fourth spine surgery.

The time goes by extremely slowly when you're alone waiting for a loved one to come out of surgery. There was no one else in the waiting room because the surgery was done at night on an emergency basis.

Finally, Dr. Oliver came into the waiting area and as always was so reassuring. He states that there was nothing seriously wrong with Morgan's spine. He removed the hardware, as he noticed that there was bursitis alongside it and he believed that the bursitis was probably the source of Morgan's discomfort.

I heard of bursitis but wasn't too familiar with it. It is a painful condition that affects the small fluid-filled sacs called bursae that cushion the bones, tendons and muscles. He said that he believed the bursitis was rubbing on the hardware and causing considerable pain for Morgan. He removed Morgan's hardware and would fit her with a brace before she left to go back to Calgary.

I wanted to believe Dr. Oliver, as he was always there for us and always listened to Morgan. I was sceptical, having gone through everything that we had. I knew that I needed to be positive for Morgan, and we had to keep looking forward.

Once Morgan was set up in the recovery room, they allowed me to go in and be with her. I was incredibly surprised about this, as I had never been in the recovery room with her before.

The screams and cries that she let out were difficult to bear, it made me thankful that I had not been in the recovery room for her other spine surgeries. The nurses worked tirelessly in the recovery room trying to adjust the medication to help Morgan fall asleep.

Just when I thought she was asleep, she let out an incredible scream and the nurses once again did their best to reassure her that everything was ok and that she would be fine.

After a few hours, we were brought to a hospital room that had three other patients in it. I asked the nurse why they would move her from the recovery room, where she was the only patient and put her in a room with three other people knowing that she had just had surgery and she told me that was just the way it was.

Scoliosis Does Not Hurt

I couldn't believe it. I knew that the first night post surgery was always tough. Her back was split open, and hardware was removed, it wasn't going to be an easy night and I felt so badly for the other patients in the room.

Occasionally, Morgan would let out a scream and I would remind her that there were other patients in the room. At this point, she could care less, not that I blamed her, it was an idiotic move to put a patient who has just come out of surgery in with 3 other patients that were fast asleep.

I was on a cot beside Morgan and every now and again she needed the nurses to help her reposition herself. This is quite normal and this being the fourth spine surgery, I was well aware of the fact that she required assistance to move herself in bed.

This one time when Morgan rang the nurses, I pretended to be asleep. When the nurse came to the bed and asked Morgan what she wanted, she said that she needed to be repositioned.

The nurse started with a lecture "you have to stop buzzing the nurse's station simply because you need to be repositioned". I popped my head up and said, "well do tell me, who should she be calling if she needs to be repositioned."

I was running on fumes. I had very little sleep over the past month being with Morgan in the hospital. I was overly stressed from the surgery and the recovery room and could only find a bag of chips to eat, which was all the food I had consumed that day. Don't mess with me, nurse.

Thankfully the next day we were headed back to the Orthopaedic Hospital. Morgan felt more comfortable there and had her own room which was a big plus.

Over the next few days as she was healing, Morgan helped with the design of her brace. She truly looked forward to wearing it because she had designed the exterior.

Before we knew it, we were headed back to Calgary. The flight was a bit difficult for Morgan due to the recent surgery, but overall, she said that she thought that her back was now better. She still had to deal with the surgical pain, but according to her, that was nothing compared to the pain she has endured over the past few years.

We got home and Morgan was gung-ho to get back to school and to sport her brace proudly. But being 16 years old, a brace is not something that she ended up liking at all. She did wear the brace to school and sometimes when I picked her up from school, she had the brace on, other times she did not.

I had no clue how many hours a day she was wearing the brace, but I was so exhausted, so totally spent from the whole ordeal, I had to let her decide for herself.

I believed that I had gained a bit of weight by sitting around that hospital all day for a month and was feeling slightly different. I couldn't tell you what it was exactly, but I felt something wasn't right.

I think back to when I had the issues with my gallbladder and the doctor at the time had some concern that I had liver cancer. I remember that I had said a prayer that conveyed that if I had to have cancer, please not when my daughter was seven years old, as she needed me.

My daughter is now 16 years old, and she still needs me, but this time I do have cancer.

www.ingramcontent.com/pod-product-compliance
Lightning Source LLC
Chambersburg PA
CBHW052319220526
45472CB00001B/184